KEEP FIT

Syd Hoare's background is in Judo – a sport demanding a high degree of all-round fitness. A former Olympic competitor, he is now one of Britain's highest graded Judomen, holding the 7th Dan red and white belt. He is a National Coach of the British Judo Association and has trained Olympic gold and silver medallists.

During his army service, he worked as a physical training instructor. He now runs a chain of gymnasiums, providing facilities and personal fitness programmes geared to a wide range of individual requirements, which are reflected in this book. His wife Sophy is a Yoga expert.

Syd Hoare is also author of *Judo* and *Self Defence* in the Teach Yourself series.

TEACH YOURSELF BOOKS

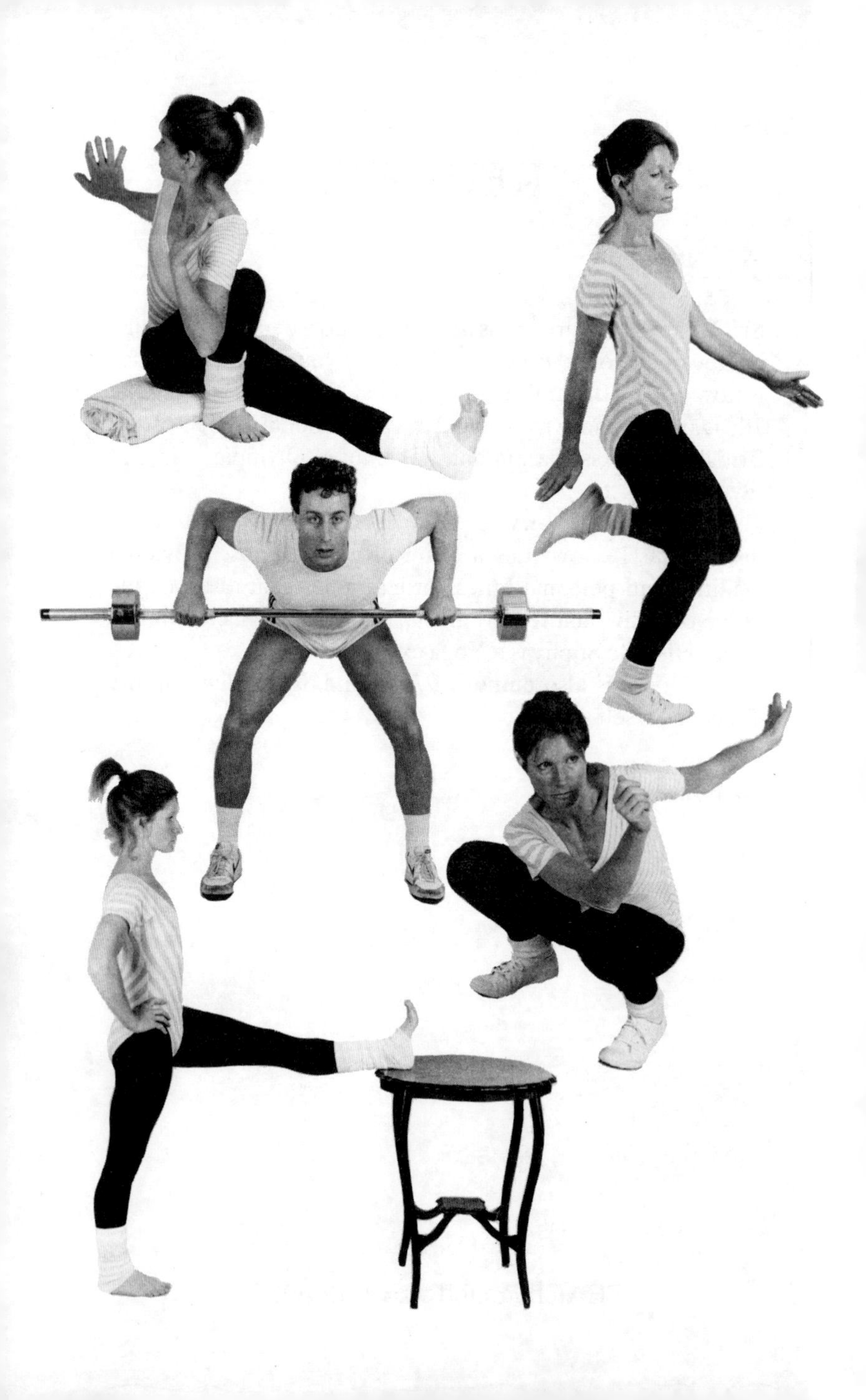

KEEP FIT

Syd Hoare

TEACH YOURSELF BOOKS
Hodder and Stoughton

First published 1986

British Library Cataloguing in Publication Data

Hoare, Syd
Keep fit.–(Teach yourself books)
1. Physical fitness
I. Title
613.7 RA781

ISBN 0 340 37626 0

Printed and bound in Great Britain
for Hodder and Stoughton Educational,
a division of Hodder and Stoughton Ltd,
Mill Road, Dunton Green, Sevenoaks, Kent,
by Richard Clay (The Chaucer Press) Ltd,
Bungay, Suffolk.
Photoset by Rowland Phototypesetting Ltd,
Bury St Edmunds, Suffolk

Contents

Introduction

Not so long ago anyone who maintained their body in good working order was labelled a fitness fanatic. The lone runner on the streets of the big cities was an object of amusement and often had to put up with derisory remarks. Suddenly this has changed. The number of runners on the streets and in the parks has increased dramatically, and sports centres and gymnasia are crowded as never before. The person who does not keep fit – whether directly by exercise, or indirectly by diet or abstention from harmful habits such as smoking – is now becoming the exception rather than the rule.

What has brought about this change? Perhaps the single most powerful cause has been the rise in illness and death from heart disease. A striking common feature of the people who suffered in this way was that they were often extremely inactive. The conclusion was drawn that these are illnesses of inactivity, and that physical activity is necessary for their prevention. This has yet to be fully established medically, though it would be difficult now to find a physician who would say that moderate exercise was bad for you.

As more and more people have taken up exercise, they have discovered that not only do they look their age or younger, but they also feel a lot better in themselves, and work and play better. Exercise has begun to be established as beneficial in its own right.

The concept of 'fitness' is an elusive one. Fitness for the athlete is relatively simple. The goal is to win, and by winning the fitness training methods are proved to be right. An athlete may only need to excel in one aspect of fitness – such as strength for the weight-lifter, or endurance for the marathon runner – and so is not so concerned with other aspects. However, the ordinary person needs a more balanced type of fitness since the goals may be varied.

This book looks primarily at the physical aspects of fitness, but also covers related subjects such as diet and relaxation.

Teaching yourself to keep fit is simple. Although much keep-fit equipment is available, little is essential, and you can exercise at most times, and on your own. Progress is easily monitored and maintained. Just a few weeks' regular exercise are needed to get you to the point where the benefits become obvious, and you will then acquire a healthy habit that will last you a lifetime.

S.R.H.

Acknowledgment

Fig. 2.1 on page 16 is reproduced with permission from Berger, R. A.: *Applied Exercise Physiology*, Lea and Febiger, Philadelphia, 1982.

1

What is Fitness?

Ask the average person what is meant by *fitness*, and the answer will probably be something like 'the ability to perform a simple physical task, such as running to catch a bus, without becoming unduly puffed or stressed'. If you were waiting at the bus stop and a friend who lived half a mile away came running up to catch the bus, and was barely out of breath, you would probably exclaim, 'Gosh, you're fit!' Of course, you would not say that if your friend was doubled up and on the verge of collapse.

The word 'fit' is used loosely in other ways. You might remark to a delivery man that he must be fit if he had just delivered a dozen heavy cases. In fact the word 'fit' may be loosely used to mean 'able to do a physical task easily'. However, for most people the one quality of the task that attracts the label 'fit' is that of endurance – physical work sustained over a period of time. Somebody who runs for five minutes to catch a bus may be described as fit, while somebody who runs for three to four hours in the marathon may be called super-fit.

The word 'fit' is also used to describe someone's appearance, as in 'You look fit'. This often refers to a lean, suntanned and bright-eyed person (who may, in fact, have little in the way of physical endurance or strength at all). And, of course, a person may remark 'I feel fit', referring to a sense of well-being and springiness.

Thus the word fit may be used to describe how easily one does a physical task, how one looks, and how one feels. This corresponds to functioning well, looking well and feeling well. Before starting to get fit it is necessary to ask yourself, indeed to be frank with yourself, about the real nature of your fitness goal. This is necessary since there are different methods to achieve the different ends.

Functional fitness

At a very specific level, functional fitness means having the physical abilities that 'fit' the task and, as the task varies, so do the physical abilities. For example, for a fireman to be 'fit' for his job, he would need very strong arms and legs for carrying heavy weights and people up and down ladders. He would not be fit for his job if he did not have such strong limbs, even if he could run a marathon.

The two main components of physical work are *strength* and *endurance*. The athlete who typifies strength is the weight-lifter, and the marathon runner typifies endurance. These two components reflect the intensity and the duration of any physical work. In addition, there are less important components allied to them such as *power* (in terms of strength and speed), and strength-endurance.

The weight-lifter who lifts more than twice his own bodyweight above his head exhibits strength. The marathon runner or the runner who runs even longer distances exhibits endurance. The shot-putter exhibits power, and the labourer who works a solid eight hours moving heavy building materials exhibits strength-endurance.

Everybody is functionally fit on some level. They have a certain amount of strength and endurance already, for without it they could not survive. Their body is a reflection of the life they lead; form follows function. That is to say, the form or shape you are is a reflection of what you do. If you are happy with the way your body copes with the day's physical demands, you will not need extra strength or endurance. If, on the other hand, the day's activities leave you exhausted, or you have no extra energy for recreational activities, then some extra physical conditioning is necessary.

Athletes know that if they want to train at any one of the components of physical work they have to do it in a particular way. That is to say, the weight-lifter does not go on marathon runs to improve his performance, neither does the marathon runner lift enormous weights. The muscles work in different ways in each activity, especially in the way that energy is produced in the muscles (see Chapter 2).

These facts do not matter that much to ordinary people unless, like firemen, they need to develop a particular requirement for their job. Probably the ordinary person will require quite a bit more endurance and perhaps a bit more strength and suppleness. These and other side-aspects of functional fitness will be looked at more closely later on.

Looking well

A number of surveys have shown that for many people the primary objective in *getting* fit is really *looking* fit. When they look in the mirror and see a lot of spare flesh, or a face that looks older than it should, they may say to themselves 'I must get fit', although it is possible that they may not need or desire any change in physical ability, as they may already be able to cope with their work and other daily activities. Probably they *do* need more activity, since overweight people are often inactive and exercise does of course help get rid of extra fat, especially around the thighs, bottom, hips and upper arms. However, achieving their goal of looking better will involve as much attention to diet as to exercise (see Chapter 12).

Looking fit and well may be achieved by a combination of eating less, reducing stress, perhaps not working quite so hard, and getting a bit more sleep, fresh air and sunshine. In other words, the necessary changes in lifestyle do not necessarily all involve increased physical activity. A person with haggard looks that are due to leading a stressful life may well make things worse with vigorous physical activity, especially if it leads to over-exhaustion. What is needed is a judicious combination of exercise and attention to diet.

Feeling well

The desire to *feel* fit is probably the second main motive in the average person's general desire for fitness. People are usually more interested in the benefits of fitness rather than the activity itself. They may wish to look and feel fit, but do not necessarily want to go out for a thirty-minute run. As with looking fit, feeling fit may be gained by a regulated lifestyle. A feeling of well-being may be gained simply by using the body, even for a few minutes. People who do yoga, for example, report a feeling of well-being. Looked at physiologically, there does not appear to be much to yoga except for some slow stretching (see Chapter 7), yet obviously just stretching the body thoroughly through its full range makes people feel good. The same may be said of weight training, where the muscles of the body are worked fairly hard against resistance, resulting in a similar feeling of well-being.

Although it may be possible to look and feel better without physical exercise, it may be quite difficult to adjust one's life in terms of stress, diet, sleep and so on. All aspects of one's life interrelate, and introducing physical exercise is one way, possibly the easiest, of changing the whole balance. This balance is also affected indirectly. Creating space in one's life, for example by cutting back on work time or learning to relax properly, gives sufficient energy and time for exercise.

Physical exercise therefore not only helps you function better, but will make you look and feel better too. It will help reduce weight, tighten the skin, and give you that extra bounce. It will also help you to sleep and eat better, and to be more aware of yourself physically, so that you will learn to recognise when you are abusing your system. It is recommended that you try a little of all the types of physical activity mentioned in these pages, from running to meditation, and eventually you should establish the right balance for your personal needs. Contrary to expectation, perhaps, men should try the exercises for suppleness, and women should try those for strength.

Full function

Having a strong and reliable body, being the right weight, and looking your age or younger is not the full story of physical fitness. The muscles and joints have a range of movement over which they must be exercised or they lose that range. This often becomes apparent in later life, with collapsing posture, and hip and back problems. A complete exercise programme should therefore contain regular sessions of stretching and twisting the body to its natural limits. Stiff muscles and joints are *not* something you have to live with. Some people claim that they have always been stiff and that nothing can be done about it. This is not so, for suppleness can nearly always be attained, although it may take a few months of patient work. Physical stiffness may also be linked with mental stiffness in some way. The expression 'stiff-necked' not only indicates a person of stubborn attitude, but probably describes a physical condition as well.

Stiffness, both physical and mental, can be worked at from two directions. Stretching exercises such as yoga (see Chapter 7) treat physical stiffness, while techniques of meditation (see page 153) treat mental stiffness. Both the physical and the mental techniques overlap in their effects, and it is wise to do both for the quickest results. A muscle may have shortened because it has been habitually used over just a small part of its range. In this case the muscle has to be patiently stretched. On the other hand a muscle may be shortened because of psychological reasons, such as anxiety. A person may be tense and not able to let go. Part of the business of being fully functioning is not only to accelerate the machine, as it were, but to throttle down and idly tick over. Techniques of meditation and relaxation help to work the body at the lower end of the activity scale. In the same way as it takes time to build up 'fitness', it also takes time to learn to relax properly and be still.

The range of function of the human body is extraordinary and is described in Chapter 2. Breathing rates may range from four breaths per minute in meditation to forty-five per minute in a young adult doing heavy physical work. The heart rate may range from fifty-three beats per minute at rest (the average for athletes) to two hundred beats per minute or more in heavy work. A working muscle may increase its output of energy by fifty times that of its resting level.

Whatever the medical reasons for taking exercise, it seems sensible that the body should be frequently taken through as wide a range of its functions as is comfortable.

Health and longevity

Health and longevity are other aspects of the full function of the body. Health is usually defined as the absence of disease. This does not really describe health however, since we can all think of someone who is not ill or diseased, but whom we would not actually call healthy. It is interesting to note that the word *health* derives from the word *whole* (+*th*), which corresponds to the *full* function of the body. Furthermore, not only must the body work fully in its several functions, but these must balance each other. The athlete who perhaps spends hours training every day to the detriment of social or spiritual life is not 'wholethy', and neither is the academic who spends hours poring over books to the detriment of both posture and physique. It is not surprising that many eminent scientists and writers report that they work better with a lifestyle that includes exercise. To be healthy is to be in tune, like the strings of a musical instrument. When they are slack the wrong notes are produced, and when overtightened they may snap. Exercise will help tune you up and the right balance of exercises will contribute to your wholeness.

Everyone desires a long and full life, and exercise has a great part to play in this. In one respect the body can be said to commence ageing from the moment it is born, although it is usual to reckon this really begins in about the middle thirties (although earlier for athletes). However, the different systems of the body age at different rates, no doubt depending upon how they are used or not used. Many people continue a very active life, both physically and mentally, well into old age. The barriers to these activities often seem to be psychological rather than physical, and when a person thinks he is too old to do something he may well be completely wrong, although, of course, too much exercise could do harm. The only way to find out if you can do something is to try it.

Whether exercise actually extends life is difficult to say. It certainly retards the visible ageing process and prevents the body from breaking down prematurely. In this respect it contributes to the fullness of life.

To be totally fit or functioning fully would appear to be quite a complicated business. However, all one really needs is to learn to listen to the body and mind, so that the proper balance can establish itself. Joggers report this growth in self-awareness and harmony, as do yoga practitioners. The vicious circle of inactivity and lack of energy is quite easily broken. One should become an artist; not the sort that produces an external work of art, but the sort which makes life itself a work of art.

How fit should you be?

It is difficult to say how physically fit you *should* be, since physical fitness is an open-ended personal condition. People vary so much that it is impossible to say how strong or durable they should be to qualify for the state called fitness. A thirty-minute run may well be more than enough for most people, but a drop in the ocean for an athlete. As we shall see in Chapter 3, it is known how long and at what rate it is necessary to run to produce changes in the heart rate, but it has yet to be proved that these changes are necessary for health. Since the human body is an adaptable organism, all one can say is that it adapts to an increased work load.

Exercise physiologists vary in their suggestions as to the length of time one should indulge in activities designed to stretch cardiovascular endurance. Kenneth Cooper of *Aerobics* fame suggests a minimum of four runs of 1½ miles (2½ km) a week, each taking about twelve minutes. Laurence Morehouse of the University of California in Los Angeles, and author of *Total Fitness*, suggests work that raises the heart rate to an optimum of a hundred and twenty beats a minute for at least three minutes, three times a week.

The problem is that the level of activity needed to protect against killer disease is so low that it is difficult to establish a control group for testing purposes.

What has to be borne in mind is that the body does not just stop when you are not taking exercise. It works all the time. Depending on what you do during the day, your heart rate may rise for a while – such as when briskly cleaning something – or you may exert some muscles to the full, as when wringing out a wet cloth. The body is in fact exercised most of the time.

The best way to assess how fit you need to be is to work forward from the condition you are in now and not aim from the outset at some hypothetical ideal. If you are overweight, or find the day exhausting or flat, or your doctor warns you against some danger of disease, start exercising and see how it affects you. If nothing happens, then try a bit more; if you feel absolutely knocked out, do less. A certain amount of perseverance is necessary since changes do not happen overnight, in just the same way that people do not become overweight overnight. Start moderately and, as you feel better or lose weight, increase gradually till you find the right level of activity. How to do this will be explored in more detail in later chapters.

When trying to establish a level of fitness one other factor needs to be taken into account. Being just fit enough is all very well, but it leaves no margin for emergencies. Sometimes you may need that extra bit of strength or endurance, for changing a flat tyre or for coping with a sudden crisis at home or work involving much longer hours. This reserve of fitness may help you to deal with these emergencies, and also protect you from illness at those moments when you could be weak or exhausted. Find your right level of activity, then add a bit more for emergencies.

Natural fitness

Apart from what your body tells you about its requirements, it is interesting to consider what the natural fitness of the body should be. The human body has evolved in response to its environment over thousands of years. About five million years ago, Australopithecus or pre-man began to stand erect. For a very long time food-gathering habits remained the same. Nuts and berries and other products of the environment were gathered from wide areas. Perhaps about one million years ago meat began to form a large part of the diet. As larger and larger animals were hunted, man, the hunter, had to move faster and for much longer periods at a time. Life, however, was not necessarily one never-ending search for food. Studies done on existing hunting-gathering tribes in remote parts of the world have shown that on average they spend two and a half days a week searching for food, and that the working day is about six hours – a fifteen hour week! However, this fifteen-hour working week is certainly quite an active one.

Perhaps the next stage was when man learnt to tame certain animals and keep them in herds, so cutting out the need to go hunting over long distances. Next, perhaps about 10 000 years ago, man learned to grow food. It is interesting to note that the agricultural stage represents only about 1 per cent of man's time on this earth. Finally man has moved to the large cities and become 'industrialised'. The working day and week is much longer than that of the hunter-gatherer, but in many cases nowhere near as active. The gradual process over the last ten thousand years or so has been for man to settle down and become less active. He is no longer out in the open looking for food on foot, and covering long distances at varying speeds.

A wide area was needed to support one hunter-gatherer but as land came to be used more efficiently, it could support an increased population. With the vast population that the world has now, there is little space for hunting-and-gathering. Unfortunately, from the exercise point of view, there is no way to turn the clock back!

Another aspect of primitive life was an irregular supply of food; sometimes there would be plenty food, and at other times very little. It was therefore most unlikely that early man was much overweight!

One can conclude that for the greatest part of man's life on this planet, the human body has evolved as a machine for gathering food, and that some physical activity that copies that search for food might well be a good thing. Long walks and runs in the country would keep us in reasonable shape, although this poses a few problems for the city dweller.

Exercise opportunities

Such is the structured sedentary existence that modern man has created for himself that the natural activity of the body now has to be slotted into a set period of time and called *exercise*. Early man with his fifteen-hour working week had no such problem. Staying alive was exercise enough, but any surplus requirements were probably met in play, dance, ritual and fighting.

Modern man now has to create exercise opportunities but they do not necessarily have to be in the strict exercise-sport category. Various aspects of our social and working lives can be utilised to make ourselves more active. It is curious that every day sees a new 'labour-saving' device on the market and that the people who buy them are probably also most in need of more physical exercise.

Given the right space, children will play for hours and get ideal exercise out of it. Some interpret play as an imitative activity in which children learn and prepare themselves for adulthood. This may well be so, but it is interesting to watch both young and not so young adults, given the same freedom and the right space, such as a warm sandy beach, express themselves in joyful activity. Although not rigidly measurable in terms of endurance, speed and resistance, play is perhaps the best form of exercise there is, simply because it is so much fun. Unfortunately, even play itself becomes structured in the progression to games and sports. Even so, games and sports can be a lot of fun, provided that one does not get side-tracked into anti-social behaviour and competitiveness. Look for opportunities to play, whether it is simply kicking a ball around in an open space or messing about in boats.

Dance is another form of physical activity found in both the most 'primitive' people of the earth and the most 'sophisticated'. Many people find they want to move to a lively rhythm – their hands and feet move instinctively to a beat without them being consciously aware of it. If you are one of those people, make a positive effort to go dancing as one of your weekly physical activities. Some dance forms are more strenuous than others, but all will get you moving, breathing, and even perspiring in the most pleasurable way.

At all times during the day there are opportunities for more physical activity. People working in office blocks can resolve to walk up stairs as often as possible. If they work on the fortieth floor they can get off the lift on the thirty-ninth and walk up the rest. Eventually they can get off the lift lower and lower down. Travel to and from work can also be used. Try catching the bus or train one stop further away and walking the remaining distance. Results from such daily extra activity may not be dramatic, but over a period of time you will find excess weight melting off, and find yourself much more lively.

Thus extra activity during the day, play, dance, games and sports, and all the forms of structured exercise can be used in different blends to change your lifestyle from a sedentary one to an active one. The only proviso with some of the spontaneous ones such as competitive play and dance is that if you are at all at risk healthwise (see page 21) you should not suddenly overdo it.

Benefits of fitness

As you exercise, a number of changes take place. On the functional side, your endurance and strength will increase, allowing you to work harder and longer with less fatigue. Your resting pulse rate will slow down at the same time as your heart volume increases. You will recover more quickly from exercise. Muscles will thicken depending on how hard you work them and excess weight will be shed. Active people tend to suffer less from coronary problems than inactive ones and, if they are afflicted, cope better. Exercise will help your bowel functions and digestion and affect your diet. Psychological problems such as depression may be helped and your mood generally will improve. The shedding of excess weight will help you to look your age or younger, and the extra physical abilities will help your sex life. Sleep may improve and niggling aches such as back-pain disappear. Several medical conditions, from diabetes to lung problems, appear to respond to physical exercise, although it is wise to consult your doctor first. A lot of research is attempting to prove that exercise is good for you, although it is obvious that your body, like any machine, must be well used to get the best out of it. At first the really unfit may have to persevere at their exercise, but gradually it will get easier and easier, and eventually become enjoyable in its own right.

2

Basic Exercise Physiology

The body consists of various systems, all of them interdependent to a greater or lesser degree. The role each system plays in the total working of the body will be more or less active depending upon the activity of the body. As one system is more active, so some of the other systems are less active. The systems are:

Skeletal
Muscular
Cardio-vascular (including lymphatic)
Neurological
Digestive
Respiratory
Genito-urinary
Endocrine

In addition, there are parts of the body which do not fit entirely into any one system, such as the skin, eyes and mammary glands. Sometimes, the first four systems are referred to as the major systems, and the second four as the minor ones, although they all play an essential part.

All of the systems are of interest to the exercise physiologists, but those of major concern are the muscular, cardio-vascular and respiratory systems, as it is in the muscles, heart and lungs that the major changes are seen during and after exercise.

The muscular system

The muscular system covers the skeletal frame of the body and accounts for approximately 40–45 per cent of the total bodyweight. Altogether there are about 640 named muscles, plus many more unnamed ones, such as those attached to each hair of the body. The muscles responsible for body movement are attached to the skeleton. Skeletal movement occurs only when the muscle contracts. For example, when the hand is moved towards the shoulder, it is the *biceps* (muscle of the front upper arm) that moves the forearm. When the hand is stretched away from the shoulder, it is the *triceps* (muscle at the back of the upper arm) that moves the lower arm. The muscles of the upper arm are attached to the bone of the lower arm, hence the movement of the lower arm when the muscle contracts. Usually muscles move in pairs, so that as one contracts the other relaxes. This can be seen in the action of the hand moving toward the shoulder or away. As the biceps contract, the triceps relax, and vice versa. As muscles contract and relax, other muscles work with them to stabilise the body as a whole, and help or modify the main muscular action.

The muscle has the capacity to vary expenditure of energy according to demand. It can apply a large force in a short time or a sustained force of longer duration. Energy output may increase by fifty times that of resting level. For this to happen, the lungs and heart must maintain a high supply of oxygen to the muscle and remove the resulting waste products. During exercise the blood flow to skeletal muscles may increase by up to twenty times that of resting flow.

Several things may happen when a muscle exerts force. It may exert force by shortening (contracting) in length or staying the same length. These actions can be seen in lifting a heavy weight, (when the muscles shorten) and in holding a weight in position (when the muscles tense but do not shorten). This is also seen when a body position is held. Normally, when a muscle contracts, the amount of force exerted differs throughout the range of movement. This can be seen when lifting a heavy weight hanging down at arm's length at your side. As you start to lift it (and the hand starts to swing up towards the shoulder) the load is moved easily, but half-way up a sticking point is felt when it is most difficult to move. At this point the muscle is contracting at 100 per cent force capacity, but not before or after that point. This is due to the leverage inefficiency of the arm at that angle. In some movements, however, the muscle may contract at 100 per cent force capacity throughout the full range of contraction. This happens when the resistance adapts to the pull of the muscle.

A muscle often exerts force by lengthening. This is when the muscle performs a 'braking' function, such as when *lowering* a heavy weight, or when absorbing the shock of landing after a jump. The force exerted in the braking action is greater than in the other types of muscular actions. For example, it is possible to lower a heavier weight than can be lifted.

The different types of muscle action are often found together in a single body movement such as jumping or throwing. The legs may be performing a braking function while the arms contract in a throwing action, and the muscles responsible for posture stay the same length. These actions are, of course, momentary and the same muscles will switch into another function at different stages of the movement. Only occasionally does the muscle contract at 100 per cent capacity throughout its full range, and that is when it is working against a constant and accommodating resistance. For example, if you were arm-wrestling with someone of equal strength, the movement pressing their hand to the table would be met *all* the way with such resistance that your arm muscles would have to work at 100 per cent force throughout the movement.

The actual measurable strength of a muscle depends on the capacity of the muscle and the leverage system (skeleton). The force capacity of a muscle can be increased with training, but nothing can be done to change the skeleton. A smaller person may often be able to lift a heavier load than someone larger, not necessarily because his muscles are stronger, but because his leverages are better, for example, his forearms and lower legs may be shorter. In general, the larger the muscles, the greater the force capacity. There are, however, some differences in quality of muscle tissue. A moderately muscled person may be very strong. An increase in muscular strength may be paralleled by enlargement of the muscle fibres, the greater recruitment of existing fibres by the nervous system and an increase in the capillary network in the muscles which increase the supply of blood and nutrients. The greater recruitment of fibres happens early in any strength training programme.

The speed with which a muscle contracts relates to the strength of the muscle when the muscle is contracting against heavy loads, but there is not such a relationship between strength and speed when the muscle contracts against light loads. In other words, a strong person can move more quickly than a weak person, especially against resistance. Note the heavy muscles of 100 metres sprinters, for example.

Within a muscle itself, there are two types of fibres – fast-twitch and slow-twitch fibres. When exercise is continued and prolonged, slow-twitch fibres show more activity than the fast-twitch fibres, as the latter are activated when the exercise is in short bursts of near maximum contraction. The muscles in untrained individuals may consist of about 40 per cent slow-twitch and 60 per cent fast-twitch fibres, but this proportion can vary enormously. Among athletes, a sprinter may have a ratio of 75:25 of fast-twitch to slow-twitch muscles, whereas a long-distance runner may reverse this proportion. It is not known whether this proportion can be greatly changed by training. The evidence seems to point to the proportion being genetic.

In all muscle tissues, the immediate source of energy is adenosine triphosphate (ATP). However, there are as many as nineteen chemical changes in the process that changes food to ATP. During work there are three main sources of ATP. When the work is explosive, of only a few seconds duration and maximum contraction, the main source of energy is ATP itself, plus that generated from CP (creatine phosphate), both stored in the muscle. For maximal work that goes beyond about ten seconds and up to about two minutes, further ATP is supplied by the breakdown of glucose of pyruvic acid (glycolysis). During this stage, lactic acid builds up to the point where the work level cannot be maintained beyond the two minute mark. If work is to continue beyond this stage ATP energy has to be produced, mainly through chemical processes for which oxygen is essential. Although oxygen contributes to energy production at *all* levels (17 per cent at the early ATP/CP stage) the proportion changes as the duration of the work increases, so that after 60 minutes of maximal exercise, oxygen contributes to 99 per cent of energy production. It is common, however, to talk of *anaerobic* processes (without oxygen, at an early stage) and *aerobic* processes (with oxygen). The switch to energy production mainly with oxygen is quite rapid. After 10 minutes exercise, aerobic processes account for about 91 per cent of energy production, and anaerobic only 9 per cent.

When the muscles contract against maximum or near maximum resistance, the limitations in performance lie in the muscles' short-term energy supply, and in the muscle fibre used (fast-twitch). For the muscles to continue to contract, there must be much less resistance and then the limitations in performance lie in the oxygen delivery systems (heart and lungs). This can be seen in the following tasks:

The 400 metre runner runs all-out for one to two minutes, and the energy production process is mainly anaerobic; on the other hand, the marathon runner paces himself to a degree (i.e. he does not sprint all the way and the muscle force exerted is nowhere near maximal), but continues for two to three hours with the energy production process 100 per cent aerobic.

The circulo-respiratory system

The cardio-vascular and respiratory systems are sometimes linked under the single term *circulo-respiratory system*. When the skeletal muscles do long and heavy work, a large supply of oxygen is needed, and the heart can increase the blood flow by almost trebling the pumping action. Not only does the increased blood flow carry more oxygen to the muscles, but the resulting waste products are carried away.

When the heart is required to pump more blood to the muscles for sustained vigorous exercise over a long period, it responds by growing bigger and increasing the amount of blood it can hold and pump in one contraction (the heart and stroke volumes). The heart-wall of an athlete may be as much as 30 per cent or more thicker than that of a non-athlete. Also an increase of 13 per cent heart volume and 25 per cent stroke volume may be seen in athletes who train in endurance events. Physical work *may* also open up more blood vessels to the heart which would help in coronary illness.

At rest, the average heart rate is about 75 beats per minute for non-trained people, and about 55 beats per minute for trained people, especially those whose work is long, sustained and aerobic. At the age of ten the average maximum heart rate is about 210 beats per minute and it drops steadily to about 165 by the age of sixty-five.

As the body starts to move from rest into hard exercise, the blood distribution to various tissues and organs changes. The amount of blood in the brain stays the same, but the flow to the skeletal muscles, skin and heart increases many times, while the flow to the abdomen and kidneys decreases. Flow is into the parts that need it, such as the muscles, and away from the parts that do not, such as the stomach. Blood movement around the body is assisted by respiratory activity, which increases venous pressure, and by the squeezing action of the contracting skeletal muscles on the veins.

Since the heart responds so quickly to muscular activity, it is a very good indicator of how much work the muscles are doing. The best indication of work is the amount of oxygen taken up during maximum work (VO_2 max). This can be difficult to measure without special equipment. However, the heart rate can be used to predict maximum oxygen uptake, albeit with a certain margin of error (12 per cent) especially at high levels of work. In other words, an increase in heart rate virtually parallels the increase in work. The prediction of maximum oxygen uptake from the heart rate must also be related to the age of the individual. For example, an athlete with a heart rate of 160 beats per minute may only be working at 65 per cent of maximum uptake, whereas a sixty-five year old with the same heart rate may be working at 95 to 100 per cent of maximum uptake.

Before improvements can be seen in heart fitness, training must reach a particular intensity, which is known as the *threshold heart rate*. Training at less than this intensity will not improve the uptake of oxygen. The intensity is related to age, and the average rate can be seen in Fig. 2.1, which assumes average cardio-vascular fitness levels. Changes in heart fitness relate not only to the intensity, but also to the duration and frequency of the exercise periods.

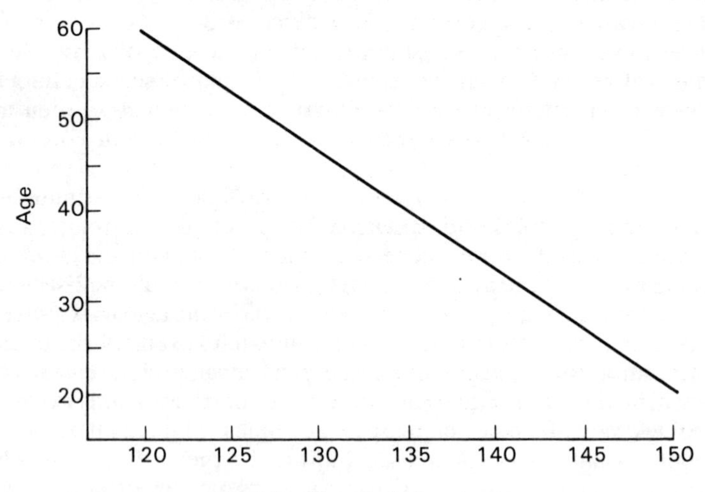

Fig. 2.1 Threshold heart rate

It is the lungs which take in the oxygen from the atmosphere for transportation to the muscles, and it is the lungs that expel carbon dioxide – the waste product derived from the chemical processes using oxygen in the muscles. The two-way process of oxygen provision and carbon dioxide removal is seen at all stages from the lungs to the actual muscle tissue. For work to continue, these processes must balance. The contraction of the diaphragm and intercostal muscles enlarges the thoracic cage, reducing the air-pressure in the lungs, which immediately causes the outside air to flow in. The muscles then relax, and the thoracic cage returns to its original size, bringing about an increase in air pressure and an immediate expiration of air. During heavy exercise, the muscles around the neck help in inspiration and the abdominal and oblique muscles aid in expiration. The lungs are similar to air-filled balloons. At rest, the contraction and expansion of the lungs during breathing stays within a limited range of movement, but as more oxygen is demanded when exercising, the balloons will contract more to expel the air, and expand more to take in more air. This increase and balance of contraction and expansion is achieved quite naturally without conscious attention being paid to breathing. The vital capacity of the lungs refers to the maximum volume of air that can be moved out of the lungs after a maximum inhalation. It is no longer believed that a large vital capacity has any relation to cardio-vascular efficiency.

After very hard work, especially anaerobic work, the breathing rate will remain high for some time. Extra oxygen is required to convert lactic acid and build up the short-term supplies in the muscles (ATP/CP). This is known as *oxygen debt.*

When exercise begins, there is a sharp rise in ventilation (breathing) which then levels off, especially with aerobic work below maximum. With heavy anaerobic work, however, the rate of ventilation increases till the end of the work.

Training also increases lung efficiency, as untrained individuals use more oxygen for breathing than trained individuals. It seems that in trained people the respiratory muscles (diaphragm and intercostal muscles) can use oxygen more efficiently. Greater elasticity in the lungs and rib cage may also enable the trained person to do more work with less oxygen.

Performance

The type of various physical exercises depends on the mix of duration and force required. High force requirement means a low duration, and vice versa. This can be seen in a number of situations. A very heavy weight can only by lifted a few times, whereas a light weight can be lifted many times. Also, it is possible to walk for several hours, run for a few hours, and sprint for only a few seconds.

More work, whether the increase is in resistance or speed, can only be done for a limited time.

Everyone has a certain force-duration profile. This can be represented by a triangle, where the peak of the triangle represents the maximum force of which the muscle is capable, and the base represents the duration for which that force can be maintained. For example, in weight training, if the most one can lift is 50 kg in one repetition, then about 45 kg can be lifted five times, 40 kg ten times, 35 kg fifteen times, 30 kg twenty times, and 25 kg twenty-five times. There is more or less a steady ratio between the weight and the number of times it can be moved. However, this changes as the external weight gets lighter, until only the body weight is moved. At this point the number of repetitions can be very high.

With training, the profile can be changed, but not necessarily proportionally. If the maximum force of which the muscles are capable is increased, the triangle has a much higher peak, but the base stays the same. That is to say, the weight-lifter gets stronger, but does not become able to run for longer periods of time. Similarly, the runner may increase the maximum running time, lengthening the base of the profile, but without affecting the maximum force used. Indeed, one marathon runner whose leg strength was tested was found to have legs of only average strength.

The middle of the force-duration profile can be changed in two ways. Either the maximum force is increased or the actual desired performance is mimicked. For example, a man who can lift a maximum of 50 kg once, is capable of lifting about 35 kg fifteen times. If he wanted to move 35 kg twenty-five times, he would have to increase his maximum force for one repetition to about 70 kg. However, he could also practise just moving the 35 kg bar until he had worked up to the ability to move it twenty-five times. This would not increase his *maximum* strength. His force-duration profile would have a bulge in it.

Another component of performance is *power*. Two men may both be able to exert a maximum force of 50 kg, but if one can do it in half a second and the other in a second, the former is more powerful. Power refers to the amount of work performed in a unit of time. Work done quickly is more tiring than the same work done slowly, because more work is done in the time. When work is explosive, as in shot-putting or high-jumping, power is the main physical component required. Since speed, especially against resistance, requires strength, power is often defined as speed plus strength. It is no coincidence that athletes in events requiring power, such as shot-putting and 100 m sprinting, are heavily muscled.

Thus, as mentioned in Chapter 1, the various physical requirements are *strength*, *power*, *strength-endurance* (sometimes known as local endurance or muscular endurance), and *stamina* (also known as aerobic endurance, cardio-vascular endurance, or circulo-respiratory endurance).

In general, improvement in each of these components is achieved by working at a level close to that of the actual performance. Maximum strength is increased by low repetitive work at about 90 per cent of maximum, and stamina is increased by working close to the desired time. For example, if you want to be able to run the full twenty-six miles of the marathon, you must come close to the desired mileage in training, and feel comfortable over this distance.

3

Starting to Get Fit

You cannot suddenly ask your body to do something it has not done for years, if at all. If you do, it will hurt, and possibly even make you sick or aggravate an existing or hidden malfunction. As the Chinese saying goes – A journey of ten thousand leagues starts with a single step. With a fitness programme, day one is a single step, day two is two steps, and so on. Approached this way, progress is gradual and pleasant, and even the ability to run marathons can be eventually acquired.

A muscle responds to *slightly* more work than it is used to by growing stronger or more durable during the subsequent period of rest. The next time it can be worked a little bit more, and it grows a little bit stronger or more durable again, and so on. The duration or the intensity of the work is gradually increased, and the body gradually adapts to the new work load. Note that it is during the periods of rest that the muscles recover and strengthen. The shock of extreme work will not stimulate muscle growth, and physical inactivity will cause the muscle to wither. If you wish to avoid an increase in muscle size, light, repetitive exercise is best.

What must be avoided is the temptation to plunge into a severe programme which may make you feel bad, and so perhaps give up. If day one of your fitness programme is well within your physical capabilities, and you walk away feeling underworked, that is fine. Day three, or even day fifteen, when you begain to feel your limits, will give you all the work you need. Try to walk away from any workout feeling pleasurably exercised and extended, but certainly not exhausted or trembling.

It is essential to ignore any physical activity that you were able to do more than two months ago, or even one month ago. It goes without saying that the middle-aged should ignore anything they could do fifteen or twenty years ago. Your fitness programme starts with you as you are now, not as you were, or as you hope to be.

Health problems

There may be hidden malfunctions of the body which exercise can aggravate. Where possible, the best screening procedure to check whether it is safe for you to exercise, is the electrocardiograph-monitored exercise test administered by an exercise technician in the presence of a doctor. Certain heart abnormalities do not show up when the heart is checked at rest. If you are under thirty-five, in good health and not suffering from any of the contraindications listed below, the chances are that exercise will present no problems. If over thirty five, you are advised to have a medical check-up before you start exercising. If any of the following conditions apply, then your doctor should be consulted first.

Heavy smoking
High blood pressure
High blood cholesterol level
Obesity
Prolonged physical inactivity
Family history of heart problems
Diabetes

If light work or exercise produces chest pains, dizziness, serious breathing difficulties or flu-like symptoms, do not punish yourself by trying to struggle on – no medals are awarded in exercising – but have a thorough check-up.

All this might sound very off-putting, but bear in mind that many cardiac rehabilitation patients are built up from very low levels of fitness to very high ones. Further information on rehabilitation is given in Chapter 11. The various problems listed above, if applicable, do not necessarily mean that there is serious cause for concern, but that you must be careful to start at the right level of intensity and duration of exercise, and to build up gradually.

Smokers and drinkers

Smokers who start to exercise, especially circulo-respiratory (stamina) work, involving the lungs, will experience certain difficulties. Inhalation of cigarette smoke causes airway resistance to increase two or threefold after several seconds. This may last for ten to thirty minutes, and as a result more oxygen is needed by the respiratory muscles. During heavy exercise, the oxygen cost of ventilation for smokers is about twice that as for non-smokers.* The same results may occur if only a few cigarettes are smoked within one hour of exercising. Exercising may help you to give up smoking, and giving up smoking will certainly help you in your exercise.

If your form of exercise requires agility, balance and coordination, alcohol should be avoided. Since even a small drink impairs these abilities, it can be dangerous to lift weights, for example, or leap around a tennis court, since you may well hurt yourself or others. Too much alcohol can, of course, damage your health, but moderate quantities may be slightly beneficial, if not taken close to exercise times.

Train-as-you-feel

When you exercise there are two people that you should listen to – your doctor and yourself. It is especially important to listen to yourself. Many people relate what they do or have or are to external factors. They say 'so-and-so has a new car, I must work harder to get one too', or 'Jones has been promoted, I must too'. In exercise too there is the danger of a creation or enhancement of a reputation or self-image. You do not have to run the mile in under six minutes or work out every day because some dynamic film star does. Neither do you have to impress friends or enemies. Simply do what feels good for you. Do not listen to your neighbour who says he runs ten miles and finishes up with one hundred press-ups before breakfast. He is probably exaggerating, but in any case those are his standards, not yours.

Some people use exercise as a rod for their own backs. They have to push themselves until it hurts. In this way they perhaps hope to discover the boundaries of the self, like latter-day ascetics. Those not so inclined should beware of taking their advice on training, or exercising with them.

Listen to what your body tells you, not only before exercise, but during it. Of course, if you are dropping with fatigue, are very tense, or have a splitting headache, do not start exercising vigorously. It may help you, but most likely it will not. There will be considerable variation in how you feel before, during and after exercise. Often you may not feel like exercising at all, only to discover that you sail enjoyably through your routine. Conversely, sometimes you cannot

* *Applied Exercise Physiology*, R. A. Berger.

wait to start, then quickly discover an underlying exhaustion that does not (or should not) allow you to do much. Sometimes the routine may be a real effort, but afterwards you feel really good, and realise that you needed it. Sometimes you feel good before, during *and* afterwards – as if on a real high – but these are the bonus workouts, and of course you can feel bad throughout, and that is when you should not have exercised.

A little perseverance is often necessary to find out what state you are in. Exercise always requires a certain amount of effort, and the idea is not to avoid this. In general, push yourself when you feel good, and take it easy if not.

This train-as-you-feel attitude was followed by the East German Waldemar Cierpinski who won the marathon in the 1976 Olympics. He said about his training 'I just run long distances until I feel I've run enough. This is usually between 15 and 20 km a day, and occasionally I'll go up to 60 km'.

People's perception of their own rate of exercise is surprisingly accurate. Research done in Stockholm* showed that a number of people who were asked to work 'somewhat hard' by their own standards, were all working at about 70 to 75 per cent of their maximum uptake of oxygen (see Chapter 2). Working 'somewhat hard' by your own standards is a good target rate. If you rate your work as 'very hard' or more, you must slow down unless you are an athlete training to that level.

Actual physical performance will vary from day to day for no apparent reason. As much as a difference of 20 per cent in maximum strength has been found in the same athlete when tested from day to day.

Fitness tests

There are a number of tests which give you an indication of how 'fit' you are. Some of these are quite strenuous and not appropriate for the really unfit. Apart from indicating your fitness, the tests also provide something against which you can monitor your subsequent progress.

A very simple, light test† checks your tolerance to exercise. The test is as follows and it is based on your pulse rate which you must learn to take. The rate at which the heart beats is a fairly accurate

* Gunnar Borg, University of Stockholm, 1971.

† *Total Fitness*, L. Morehouse and L. Gross (Granada 1977).

guide to how hard the body is working (see Chapter 2) and it can be used to tell you whether what you are doing is not enough, just right, or too much. The pulse rate can be taken at the wrist (palm side just below the fleshy base to the thumb) or at the neck. Place your hand as if to seize the adam's apple, then carefully push the index finger and thumb deeper into the neck beside it. You should then pick up a strong beat. Since the thumb itself may give a beat, use the index finger to take the count. What you will need to ascertain is the rate at which the heart is beating per minute. However, if you count for a whole minute you can get a confusing reading, as the pulse rate can drop quite a bit in a minute if it has previously been working at a high rate. The ideal way to get a quick accurate check is to count the pulse for ten seconds, then multiply that figure by six to get the minute rate. The pulse should be taken immediately after the exercise.

Since the average pulse rates for rest, standing and work are known, the following light test gives you a good idea of where you stand and how your body tolerates the work. There are four stages.

1 Checking your resting pulse

Your *basal* pulse rate can be found by checking it first thing in the morning before you get out of bed. This basal pulse rate is often used by athletes. A record of the rate is kept for two or three weeks, then the average is worked out. From then on the basal pulse rate is used to give an indication of whether the day ahead can be used for a lot of intensive work or just a tick-over. If it is average or below, the day ahead is a work day, and if it is significantly above average, the athlete should take it easy.

However, for this test we need to find the resting rate which comes close to the normal condition of wakefulness. Since many things may accelerate your pulse, it should be taken on a day when you feel quite well, and not close to exercise, a meal, smoking, or coffee. Sit down and rest for a few minutes, do not talk or cough but just stay still. After a few minutes of quiet sitting, consciously try to relax – sink into your chair, slow your breathing, and let your muscles sag. Now take your pulse rate. It should be less than 100 beats per minute. If it is not, and you can think of no possible reason, check with your doctor. If it is below 100, move to the next stage.

2 Standing pulse rate

Stand quietly, at ease, for one minute. Do not move around or fidget or hold yourself rigidly to attention. Gently check your pulse rate. If it is twenty beats or more higher than your resting rate, check with your doctor. A rise of ten beats per minute when changing from sitting to standing is quite normal. Move to the next stage.

3 Step test
First find a suitable step between 7 and 12 inches (18 to 30 cm) in height. Next look at the chart in Fig. 3.1, and read across from your bodyweight to the column representing the height of your step. The number indicated will be the number of times you will have to step up and off the step in one minute. Step on and off the step or bench

Bodyweight (kg/lb)	*Height of step (cm/in)*					
	17·5/7	20/8	22·5/9	25/10	27·5/11	30/12
55/121	30	30	30	30	30	30
65/143	30	30	30	30	20	20
75/165	30	30	30	20	20	20
85/187	30	30	20	20	20	20
95/209	30	20	20	20	20	20
105/231	20	20	20	20	20	20

Fig. 3.1 The step test

for one minute at the required rate, then take your pulse rate immediately. If you experience any difficulties during the stepping stop immediately, and if your pulse rate is 120 or more per minute, check with your doctor. If it is less than 120 beats per minute, step up and down for another minute at the same rate and take your pulse again. If it goes over 120, stop the test, but if it is under that figure proceed for a third and final minute at the same rate on and off the step. Check your pulse rate as before – it should be under 120. Note that this stage comprises three bouts of stepping if the pulse rate is low enough.

4 Recovery test
Having completed the third bout of stepping, sit down and rest for one minute, then take your pulse rate again. The difference between your pulse rate at the end of the stepping and one minute later should be no less than ten beats. That is, it should be under 110 beats per minute.

This is a very light test, and if your pulse rate goes over 120 at any time, you are not in very good physical shape. That is not to say that there is necessarily anything wrong with you, but you should get yourself checked out before you start. If at any time during the test you have difficulties, or if you fail to meet the various pulse requirements, then stop doing the test. It has then told you all you need to know.

The twelve-minute distance test

Those who know they are in reasonable condition should try the twelve-minute distance test*. First you need to be able to measure the distance you will cover. A running track is ideal, but otherwise use your car milometer on a long stretch or clear circuit. All you have to do is go as far as you can in twelve minutes running (or walking if necessary). At the end of twelve minutes, work out how far you have covered. The chart below will indicate your fitness category, which depends on your age and sex as well as the distance covered.

Obviously with this type of test you will have to push yourself fairly hard, but do not do it to the point of collapse.

Recovery test

The following test is concerned with your recovery from exercise. As you get fitter, so you will recover more quickly from exertion.

After a set task of your choice, such as a one mile run, immediately record your pulse rate for fifteen seconds and multiply by four to give the rate for the minute. Rest for a minute and a half, then record your pulse rate for a further fifteen seconds, again multiplying by four to give the minute rate. The test must always be a smooth quick sequence of run-check-rest-check, with no gaps in between. To gain a score from these figures, deduct the second slower figure from the first.

If your pulse rate immediately after the mile was 150 beats per minute, and a minute and a half later it was 100 beats per minute, then your score would be fifty. As you get fitter your pulse rate will slow down more quickly. The idea is to achieve as high a score as possible. After a few months of running, your pulse rate after a minute and a half's rest might be 90, giving you a recovery score of 60. This recovery rate score does not contrast you with other people, but simply tells you whether you are recovering more quickly, which is consistent with increasing fitness.

* *Aerobics*, K. Cooper.

MEN

Fitness Level	*Ages 13–19*	*20–29*	*30–39*	*40–49*	*50–59*	*60 Plus*
Very Poor	<1·30	<1·22	<1·18	<1·14	<1·03	<0·87
Poor	1·30–1·37	1·22–1·31	1·18–1·30	1·14–1·24	1·03–1·16	0·87–1·02
Fair	1·38–1·56	1·32–1·49	1·31–1·45	1·25–1·39	1·17–1·30	1·03–1·20
Good	1·57–1·72	1·50–1·64	1·46–1·56	1·40–1·53	1·31–1·44	1·21–1·32
Excellent	1·73–1·86	1·65–1·76	1·57–1·69	1·54–1·65	1·45–1·58	1·33–1·55
Superior	>1·87	>1·77	>1·70	>1·66	>1·59	>1·56

WOMEN

Fitness Level	*Ages 13–19*	*20–29*	*30–39*	*40–49*	*50–59*	*60 Plus*
Very Poor	<1·0	<0·96	<0·94	<0·88	<0·84	<0·78
Poor	1·00–1·18	0·96–1·11	0·95–1·05	0·88–0·98	0·84–0·93	0·78–0·86
Fair	1·19–1·29	1·12–1·22	1·06–1·18	0·99–1·11	0·94–1·05	0·87–0·98
Good	1·30–1·43	1·23–1·34	1·19–1·29	1·12–1·24	1·06–1·18	0·99–1·09
Excellent	1·44–1·51	1·35–1·45	1·30–1·39	1·25–1·34	1·19–1·30	1·10–1·18
Superior	>1·52	>1·46	>1·40	>1·35	>1·31	>1·19

Key: < = less than; > = more than
Distances shown are given in miles

Fig. 3.2 The twelve-minute distance test

How to exercise

Any single workout should consist of a warm-up period, the main phase of the workout, and then a warm-down or tapering-off period. Warming up has several functions. Firstly, the muscles are literally warmed up, as exercise will raise the body temperature a few degrees and this helps the muscles to work more smoothly and efficiently. Secondly, a good warm-up helps to avoid muscle and joint injuries. It is not advisable to rush headlong into exercise, especially as you get older. How long you should spend warming up varies from individual to individual, but you should do it to the point of sweating.

Part of the warm-up should consist of a few separate stretching exercises (see Chapter 7). Most people who are just exercising and not competing in an athletic event need only do a few stretches, then a slow light imitation of the main phase of their workout. For example, joggers need only begin with a few calf and ham-string stretching exercises, then start jogging very slowly and lightly until they start to warm up, then they can increase their pace and get into their main workout. Your clothing and the climate will obviously affect your warm-up time, so the general rule is start gently for a few minutes, and speed up as you start to sweat or feel quite warm.

The main phase of the workout will proceed as planned, or for as long as you feel good. However, when you feel you have done enough, you should not stop abruptly. The heart pumps out the blood and your working muscles help pump it back again when they contract. If you stop suddenly, the heart has to work harder, so at the end of your run, you should gradually slow down, walk for a minute or two, and then sit down. Never stop abruptly and remain standing or you will feel very dizzy.

Unless you are in a cold wind do not immediately cover up after exercising. Your body will need to cool down and this is not helped by putting on extra layers of clothing. Stay as you are until you feel a slight chill and the need to put on extra clothes.

For those new to exercise (and those coming back to it after a break) it is important to build up gradually. This is known as *progressive overload*. A slightly more intense or longer bout of physical work than usual will cause the body to adapt to meet the extra demands made upon it, providing it has had sufficient nutrition and rest. However, the extra demands must be slight as the body cannot be shocked into adaptation. Given the right nutrition, rest, and a gradually increasing workload the body will adapt (grow stronger or more durable) almost indefinitely. Progress will not necessarily be smooth, but over a period of weeks and months an improvement will be seen. Adaptation unfortunately works the other way. If you do nothing for a week or more, you will start to lose what you have gained. If you are forced to give up exercise for a month or more, do not re-start at your former level, but begin at a much more comfortable lower level, and start to overload again gradually.

When to exercise

Ideally, when you exercise should depend on how you feel. At certain times of the day or year you will feel energetic, and it is wise to take full advantage of these times. It is interesting to note that many animals hunt in the early morning and late afternoon. The period in the middle of the day is a period of relative inactivity, and many people feel similarly inactive during this time. The best time to exercise is in the morning. Not only are you physically fresher at this time, but your will-power is stronger. As the day wears on, the vital decision to start exercising gets progressively harder to make.

Most people have to work, so it is not easy to exercise just as the mood takes them. Their exercise has to fit round their work hours. Exercise early in the morning before work can be extremely refreshing, but except for the iron-willed few it is rather impractical. The body takes a while to wake up, and suddenly plunging it into exercise may be a bit of a shock. However, it may be worth trying for a week or two, especially in summer, to see how your body takes to it.

Exercise taken after work has to take into account the evening meal and bedtime. You must not exercise too soon after a meal, which probably means that you will have to exercise before the evening meal. Since exercise tends to depress the appetite for a while, this may be useful for those trying to lose weight. If the exercise is taken too close to bedtime the body may be so stimulated that it has difficulty falling asleep.

Regularity of exercise

As much as possible, a certain regularity is necessary for your workouts. Regular progressive overloading of the body will build it up, but since you start to lose what you have gained after a few days of inactivity, irregular workouts may mean negligible progress. Three sessions a week is ideal, and twice a week is the minimum.

Youngsters may be able to cope with a single workout a week and get something out of it but older people may find it too much of a shock to the system. However, this will depend on what else they do during the week, and an active older person may find a single workout a week beneficial.

If you exercise as the mood takes you, or according to your bio-rhythms as some might describe it, you will probably be a lot more active in the summer, and also at weekends. Use the summers to get fit and lean, but do not then lapse into inactivity during winter. Try to maintain the momentum of the summer's activity to carry you through the winter. If your weekends are physically active, try to include at least one session in the middle of the week to achieve a rough regularity.

It is wise to be realistic about regularity of exercise. It is easy to work out a strict regime, but extremely difficult to stick to it. Inertia, colds, fatigue, holidays, and extra work will all conspire to stop you for various periods. Once having lapsed from your workouts it is fatal to stop altogether. Realise from the start that your exercising will probably be spasmodic, accept that fact, and be prepared to continue on that basis. Exercise is partially an acquired state of mind, which you do not lose so quickly. Getting back into a routine after a few week's break may not be as difficult as you imagine. Remember to resume with a gentle workout. After a longish lay-off even a short five-minute jog around the block may be enough to get you back in the mood.

An exercise calendar is a great help to the spasmodic exerciser. Find a calendar which has space against the different days to write in, and keep a record of what you do. Choose one that shows the whole month at a glance and hang it up in a prominent position. If you do not use such a calendar, you may find it amazing how many days can drift by without you doing anything, so this is very important.

Temperature

Exercising in the heat, especially humid heat, presents one or two problems. Although the body heats up at the start of exercise, it only rises a few degrees and then stabilises. In a very hot climate the body will have to work harder to maintain its increased exercise temperature. If you exercise regularly in such a climate then you will have adapated to the extra work. However, if you suddenly plunge into a workout on a hot day (while on holiday for example), then bear in mind that your regular workout will be harder on the body.

It takes about two weeks to acclimatise properly to heat. When exercising in hot conditions special care must be taken to replace fluid and salt lost through sweating.

There are two conditions to watch for – heat exhaustion and heat stroke. The symptoms of heat exhaustion are a rapid, weak pulse and a cold and clammy skin. Rest and fluid intake are required. The symptoms of heat stroke are a hot and flushed skin, usually dry, a high body temperature, and sometimes delirium, and medical attention is needed.

Exercising in the cold is much less of a problem. Adequate clothing must be worn to maintain the correct body temperature. When it is extremely cold the amount of clothing worn may interfere with the ability to exercise (see overleaf on clothing).

Fluid loss through sweating must be replaced. If you know that you are going to sweat a lot, drink a cupful of fluid before you start, and take regular mouthfuls during your exercise. This applies especially to those indulging in long bouts of exercise such as marathon running. The best results are obtained when fluid intake equals fluid loss.

Where to exercise

The easily-motivated fitness addict has no difficulty in finding places to exercise. Even prisoners in solitary confinement find it possible to put together a few exercises to keep themselves ticking over. However, those new to exercise may find it a problem. There are obvious places to go such as sports centres, gymnasiums and health clubs. Some people are reluctant to use such places, believing that they are full of lithe, suntanned, superfit people and so they will stand out as overweight and unfit. It is advisable to look around, as the majority of people using such centres are by no means superfit, and it should be possible to find a place where you can slide comfortably into the background. Try to look the part – buy track suit and proper shoes, and go with a friend. It is possible to exercise alone, at home or in a local green space, but experience shows that many find it difficult on their own and give up. Dressing for the occasion and going to a sports centre with a friend or training partner makes it a lot easier to sustain.

Clothing

It is important to be comfortable when you exercise. The most important item will be what you wear on your feet, especially if jogging. There are specialist shoe-shops which are well worth trying. Running magazines are a good source of information about running shoes and where to buy them. Good shoes will avoid chaffing and injuries, and will also make you feel like moving. Do not put up with poor footwear, or you will certainly regret it.

If running in the cold, wear several thin layers rather than one thick one, and if running in the heat wear clothing made of material such as cotton, which allows the sweat to evaporate. Shorts, vest or track-suits must not be so tight that repeated movement chafes the skin. Large-busted women may find specially constructed exercise bras are useful, and these are available from specialist running shops.

Some people over-dress when exercising. It is not uncommon to see someone jogging in midsummer wearing a thick tracksuit, with towel tucked in round the neck and some form of head covering. Such people suffer from two illusions. The first is that they have to dress well to stop catching cold, and the other is that profuse sweating is good. Since exercise soon warms you up, the only extra clothing you may need on a cold day is something to stop the wind penetrating. Sweating is a device for cooling down the body. Although the scales will show a few kilos weight loss after vigorous exercise, this will be entirely sweat loss, which must and will be replaced for the body to function properly. A water loss of only 2 per cent can impair both the circulatory and thermoregulatory mechanisms of the body. Since sweating usually accompanies exercise, there is some real weight loss as the exercise will burn up so many calories. However, weight lost through sweating in a sauna, for example, is an illusory loss.

Only in one respect does over-dressing or extra heat have any effect on weight loss, and that is because the body must work harder to stay cool. However, it is easier to make the body work harder by doing more exercise, for instance by running a few minutes longer, under much more comfortable conditions.

Choosing a fitness programme

Those keen to start a fitness programme may feel confused at this point. There are several aspects to fitness, different ways of achieving the same end, a number of overlapping activities, and, of course, individual preferences to be taken into account.

The five main problems – excess weight, lack of stamina, weakness, stiffness, stress or tension – are all helped to a greater or lesser degree by most of the activities in the four main groups of exercises – jogging (including swimming, cycling and walking), callisthenics (keep fit, aerobic dance, and so on), weight training (free weights and with resistance machinery), and yoga (stretching, relaxing, and meditation).

However, for each fitness problem there is a best activity, some second-best activities, and other activities which have an indirect or slight effect. A lot depends on how the activities in the second and third groups are done. Callisthenics, for example, can be a fast and vigorous dance-based activity, or a slow, gentle sequence of movements; and weight training can be a slow muscle-building grind or a fast, workout which makes you sweaty and breathless.

Below is a brief outline of the various fitness problems and recommendations to combat them. In addition there is a chart (Fig. 3.3) which shows at a glance which kind of activity is best for which problem. This chart can be used in two ways to start the construction of your fitness programme. First, decide which are *your* fitness problems and goals, then check to see which activities will help. For example, if your problem is lack of stamina, then look at the first column, and you will see that jogging or similar activities are the most beneficial, and callisthenics and weight training can also be useful. You can also use the chart to check which problems are helped by any particular activity. For example if you look at the column marked *Yoga*, you will see that this kind of activity will help you combat stiffness and tension.

Even this rough guide may be too clinical an approach for many.

	Jogging	*Weights*	*Yoga*	*Callisthenics*
Lack of stamina	A	B		B
Weakness	B	A	B	B
Stiffness			A	B
Tense	C		A	C
Overweight	A	B	C	B
Underweight		A		B

Key: A = Most benefit B = Some benefit C = Indirect effect.

Fig. 3.3 Constructing a fitness programme

Some may say, 'Look, I just want to get a bit fitter, or lose a little weight or feel a bit more lively, so what's the best thing to do?' The simplest answer is walking or running, or both, two or three times a week. The essential thing is to get started, so if you do not want to make the whole thing too complicated, just follow your inclination, and try something that you think you might like. The more things you try, the greater the likelihood of finding something that is suitable. You may find you enjoy something you had never tried before, so do not dismiss any form of exercise as unsuitable. For example, there are very few forms of exercise that a woman cannot do that a man can. For some of the harsher exercises which involve explosive movements and abrupt changes of direction, some evidence suggests that women are liable to muscle and tendon tears unless they prepare themselves thoroughly, but with preparation, a woman can make herself as much as fifty per cent fitter than the average male, in terms of stamina. However, read this book through first so that you understand fitness properly, and are able to avoid any health hazards.

Problems of being unfit

Overweight

Weight is reduced by eating less or being more active, or best of all, doing both at the same time (see Chapter 12). Most energy is used up in continuous activities, such as jogging and swimming. The longer and the more often you do them, the greater the fat loss. Callisthenics and weight training are second-best activities, although it depends how vigorously they are done. Yoga has an indirect effect in that it may reduce the need to overeat.

Lack of stamina

The best activities for stamina are in the jogging category. Callisthenics and weight-training are not as good unless done vigorously and continuously. A check of your pulse rate during each of these activities will show how they compare. Work out two or three times a week.

Weakness

The activity you choose to correct weakness depends on how strong you want to be. The most direct way of increasing strength is using weights or resistance machinery of the type found in a gym, two to three times a week. However, sufficient strength for everyday activities can be gained from callisthenics and even yoga. Many of the activities in the jogging category only strengthen the legs, although swimming gives moderate all-round strength.

Stiffness

Stiffness is best treated with yoga-type stretching, done at least twice a week. Stretching exercises done in a callisthenics class may be effective provided that they are done slowly and not forced. To the average person stiffness may not seem be a problem, as they may not be aware of their stiffness. You can test your own suppleness by checking if you can do the following: tie your shoelaces; twist round when driving to look behind; if a woman, do up your own bra and dress zips; wash your back; squat or kneel comfortably; arch up in the prone position, as when lying on a beach; and spread the legs wide to the side, as in the splits.

Tension and stress

Yoga, relaxation and meditation are the most direct ways of dealing with stress. If you wish to relieve stress, short spells of yoga and relaxation can be done daily. It may be possible to meditate every day, but care must be taken that the practice does not make you 'heady' or too introspective (see page 157). Relief can also be obtained from any *enjoyable* physical workout. Arduous workouts may make the problem worse.

Underweight

This is not usually a problem, except for those suffering from anorexia nervosa. Those who want to put on weight or change their shape will find that the best way to increase muscle size is to use weights and gym machinery, two or three times a week. Exercise of any sort should stimulate muscle growth, especially in men.

The older person

Older people may feel that they have a fitness problem in that they are aware of their physical abilities declining with age. The problem is not so much the decline but the belief that there is a problem. The body will respond well to exercise at virtually any age. The older person can do many activities provided he or she carefully builds up to it, for example, some people in their sixties can run marathons. However older people should check with their doctors before undertaking unaccustomed physical activity.

Walking and swimming are good ways to begin exercising, and yoga is ideal for correcting increasing stiffness and bad posture. A light callisthenics class or light gym work will help to maintain strength, or even increase it.

4

Stamina

Stamina or endurance, especially circulo-respiratory endurance, is the main component of fitness. This is work that is of low muscle force involving large muscle groups for a lengthy period of time. Often this type of work is called *aerobic* endurance, indicating that it is work of a duration and intensity that requires mainly oxygen-combusted energy. Examples of aerobic activities are running, cycling and swimming. A typical runner is long-muscled (not chunky like a weight-lifter), without excess weight, and with an efficient heart and good lungs.

Assuming that you have checked your fitness level according to the advice in Chapter 3 and are ready to start, how should you set about it? With any programme of exercise there are three main things to consider: frequency, duration, and intensity/speed. Only one of these three is a rigid requirement, and that is frequency. As mentioned in Chapter 3, you must try to do a minimum of two sessions a week. Three times a week is ideal, but more than that is not really necessary. Frequency is essential because you start to lose what you have gained after a few days' inactivity. You must try to keep adding to, or at least maintaining what you have gained. Getting out will be your major effort in exercising, not so much what you do when you are out.

How long you should exercise, and at what rate are not rigidly laid down. The reason for this is two-fold. Firstly everyone has different goals and starts out at different levels. Age, weight, unhealthy habits such as smoking, and the day-to-day fluctuations in your physical condition, make it impossible to lay down rigid targets. Secondly, your body will let you know when it has done enough. The training rule is: exercise as you feel, and if you feel fine make it 'fairly hard'. 'Fairly hard' refers to your own scale of perceived effort, ranging from *light*, through *moderate*, *fairly hard*, and *hard*, to *very hard*. On days when you feel below par, still train as you feel, but do less. Do not worry about only doing a little as long as you make it up on the days when you feel good.

Whether you have established some sort of fitness category (as in the tests in Chapter 3) or not, start your exercise programme with a session of light intensity and short duration. It does not matter if you come back from it feeling as if you have done nothing. After a few outings you will be getting close to your existing training limits (i.e. it will seem fairly hard). This also applies when you come back after a few weeks' break.

With a train-as-you-feel programme, it is necessary to keep some record of your achievements. Write down on your training calendar how long the session took, and what distance you covered. Also keep a record of your bodyweight and measurements. Over a period of a couple of months you will see your exercise sessions lengthening, weight decreasing, and certain measurements changing. Providing you exercise to the level which *you* regard as 'fairly hard', you are bound to see an improvement. This level is not a fixed level. As you get fitter, the level will rise, and you will naturally have to do more to achieve it (although it will feel the same).

The duration of your exercise session will vary according to how you feel. On a bright sunny day, when you are well rested, you will naturally feel like doing more, and this is the time to do more. Over a period of time, experience will tell you how much to do. For example, on a good day you might go on to do hours of aerobic activity, but then take a few days to recover from the resulting fatigue. If, however, you know that the next day is going to be a hard-working day, when you must pace yourself by not doing so much, even though you are capable of it.

For those who exercise to avoid coronary problems and the like, it is important to learn how to exercise as you feel, and listen to your own body. You cannot drive yourself through warning symptoms such as chest pain. One of the risk factors associated with heart and other problems is stress. Those who set themselves a rigid, severe programme of *x*-miles a day, and drive themselves relentlessly to achieve that, are really expressing their stress in a different form. In the long term very few rigid programmes are maintained.

Progression

There are a number of ways of structuring any one exercise session in order to avoid over-exertion and staleness. The very unfit will have to work towards a continuous period of exercise by starting with short periods of work and rest. For example, if badly out of shape you may have to start with one minute of work followed by three minutes of rest, followed by one minute of work and three minutes of rest, and so on. The length of the periods of work and rest, and the duration of the total exercise period, are each determined by how you feel. Gradually, the periods of rest are shortened to one minute; then the pattern can be changed to two minutes work followed by three minutes rest, and so on. For example:

Stage	*Work (mins)*	*Rest (mins)*
1	1	3
2	1	2
3	1	1
4	2	3
5	2	2
6	2	1
7	3	3
8	3	2
9	3	1
10	4	3

At some point, even the unfit will feel like moving on to one continuous period of work. Aim for a period of about twelve to fifteen minutes. This is best tried when the total of your work periods in the work–rest sessions exceeds fifteen minutes. At about stage twelve, if proceeding as above, you may have done four or five four-minute work periods interspersed with rest periods. The total work would have been sixteen to twenty minutes, so there should be no problem shifting to a lower continuous work period of twelve to fifteen minutes. This is the way a very unfit person would built up a workout. Of course, somebody with a better level of fitness might start at five minutes of work and a minute or two of rest repeated three or four times, and then switch quickly to a continuous period of work. Many people will be able to start with twelve minutes or more of continuous work, and might want to know how long they should run (or swim, and so on). The answer is, as before, to run for as long as it feels good. What you do is what you become. If you run for twenty minutes, you then have twenty minutes of circulo-respiratory endurance. You can build up to the marathon if that feels good for you.

Once you are a couple of months into your routine and feel very comfortable with what you do, you may want to change the pace of your routine. This can be done by alternating between slow and fast periods of activity. For example, if you go out running, you could run fast or sprint between every fifth lamppost or any other convenient marker. You could simply run faster or as fast as you can exactly when you feel like it. When you run faster, of course, you push yourself closer to your maximum limit, so it is necessary to have some training background behind you. It is not for the unfit.

There is quite a different feeling experienced when running all-out. The body feels totally used, which it does not necessarily feel when jogging or running at moderate speed for a period of time.

To summarise the principles of stamina work: make sure you go out two or three times a week. Record what you do – the length and intensity of the session depends on how you feel. If starting from a low level of fitness, break it up with small periods of rest and work. After a couple of months of regular sessions, put in the occasional fast burst.

Walking and running

The easiest way to work on your stamina is to go out for a walk or run or a combination of both. Depending on how fit you are or how fit you feel, you have a choice of speed in this type of activity. At the lowest level, there is a slow walk, followed by a normal speed walk, then a brisk walk. As you start to pick up speed, you can jog, run, or sprint. A jog is a very slow run. Some would say that a mile covered in under eight minutes is running, and anything slower is jogging. A slow walk would not appear to demand much stamina, but all exercise is relative. To someone recovering from a heart attack, it is an excellent way of building up stamina (see Chapter 11).

Walking is an excellent form of exercise and, if practised regularly, will bring many of the benefits of fitness including a gradual loss of excess weight. Obviously walking up hills or mountains is more strenuous than walking on flat city streets, and also more healthy.

The great advantage of walking and running is that they are so simple. No special area is required; in fact you can start walking or running the moment you step out of your front door. It is also the closest you will get to becoming a food-gathering machine like the early hunter-gatherer was. The right footwear is all you need to start (see page 32), and no special technique is required, just walk as you normally do. The usual technique of running is to land on the heel, and roll on to the toes. It is only when sprinting that you will be running on the balls of the feet. Some aches and pains are unavoidable to start with. However, if you start at a low level and work steadily up, and work as you feel, there is no reason why aches and pains should bother you unduly. Those new to jogging may find their leg strength a limiting factor as much as their lack of puff! Try building up leg strength with a gradually increasing number of knee bends (see page 95), or if you have access to a gymnasium, with squats, calf raises, leg extensions and leg curls (see pages 72–4).

Swimming

This is an excellent form of developing stamina, with many other advantages. The water supports the weight of the body, thus avoiding the occasional jarring motion of running, and it is very relaxing. Not only does it develop stamina, but also strength. Pulling hard through the water develops strength in a particular way. The motion tends to be at a constant velocity (that is the water slows the motion), which means that the muscles work fully throughout their range. Swimmers report not only a feeling of relaxation, but increased suppleness as well. Of course it is not quite as easy to go swimming as to go running, as facilities are more limited, and in the cold weather you may not particularly feel like it. However, it is well worth making the effort, and as with walking and running, the major requirement is to get started. Once you are at the pool, swim for as long as you feel like, and do a variety of strokes. As you change the strokes, you change the intensity of the exercise. Crawl, backstroke and breaststroke demand roughly equal effort at slow speeds. At higher speeds, backstroke and breaststroke are marginally more strenuous than the crawl. Most strenuous of all is the butterfly. It is well worth learning to do all the strokes since this gives the body more of a complete workout by using it in different actions.

Cycling

Cycling is another form of aerobic activity. The work is mostly light, and it is continuous. Cycling in big cities may be somewhat dangerous, although it is possible to pick a time such as early morning when it would be quite pleasant to cycle around empty streets. Alternatively, a long ride in the countryside at the weekends is a very pleasant way of exercising. The heavier the bike you ride, the harder you have to work, so it is worth buying a lightweight modern bicycle. If you are going to spend some time in the saddle, make sure it is a comfortable one. Also have wind-and waterproof clothing, as you will feel rain and wind more when travelling at speed.

Other stamina activities

Any activity that raises the pulse rate to a threshold minimum of about 75 per cent of the maximum and keeps it there for a while is stamina work (find your theoretical maximum by deducting your age from the figure of 220). Obviously many activities could fit into this category, for example, sports such as squash, tennis, soccer and handball, and also vigorous dancing. You need to make sure that you do not stop for any appreciable length of time during the activity, otherwise your average pulse rate for the period will fall below the threshold rate (see page 16).

Apart from the activities listed above, there are a number of exercise machines and other pieces of equipment that are ideal to develop stamina. These can be used indoors or kept at home, which avoids the necessity of going somewhere to exercise. They are also very useful when the weather prevents outdoor work, for example, during the winter.

Exercise bicycle

One of the most useful pieces of equipment is the exercise bicycle. You are advised to buy a good quality one with equipment to adjust the resistance, and show the speed and distance travelled. The exercise bike is not the most exciting piece of equipment, but it is extremely convenient. The exercise can be measured exactly in terms of distance, speed and resistance, and it is very easy to slot in several minutes of exercise per day. Your legs will ache at first, but you will quickly get used to the exercise.

Rowing machine

A similar piece of equipment is the rowing machine. Compared with the bicycle, this equipment works many more muscles, and so is much more strenuous. Resistance can be adjusted on these machines, but speed or distance travelled is not indicated.

Motorised treadmill
The motorised treadmill is a much more expensive piece of equipment. It can be adjusted for incline and speed, and can give you a very accurately measured run or walk.

Skipping rope
The training that boxers do is excellent for improving stamina. The skipping rope is cheap to buy, but it does take a while to get used to it. To start with, spend a few minutes a day practising the technique. At first the rope may catch your feet at almost every turn. Gradually, however, you will improve your timing, and need only jump one or two inches clear off the ground. There is a tendency to make enormous leaps in the beginning, which quickly proves very tiring. Aim for economy of effort in the jumping. Start with slow jumps with both feet, bringing the rope forward over your head. As you get used to it, speed the rope up, and do not jump so high. Next try two hops on one foot, followed by two hops on the other foot and eventually hop from foot to foot. It will not take too long before you can skip in a relaxed economical manner for several minutes.

Punch-bag
The punch-bag can also be used for stamina work. You will need a pair of gloves to protect your hands. If you have never punched a bag before, take care not to sprain your wrist or thumb. Clench your fist, and place the thumb outside the fist, so that the top joint of the thumb touches the middle finger between the first and second joints. When the bag is punched, there should be a straight line from the knuckles to the elbow, otherwise you may sprain your wrist if the hand buckles in. When using the bag for training, move lightly round it, moving in to the bag to make a smart left-right punch, then move out again. As you get used to punching, the pattern of blows can be changed, punching more times with each hand before moving out and also varying the target from top (head) to middle (stomach). This work can be intensified by punching harder or faster, or for longer periods. A combination of skipping and punch-bag work works the body evenly, giving you spring in the legs, and condition in the upper body.

Stair or bench
If money and training opportunities are limited, stamina work can be done on a step of some kind, such as a stair or bench. Simply step on and off it at a moderate to fast rate. Work out how many steps are

equivalent to one storey, then see how many storeys you would have climbed in your workout.

Callisthenics

Simple callisthenics can, of course, be used for stamina work. However, they must be done quickly with little or no rest in between, to get the pulse rate and breathing rate up and keep them high (see Chapter 6 for a detailed treatment of callisthenics).

The particular aspect of fitness on which you are working is your endurance. You must *endure* the activity, and make yourself *durable*, for a *duration* of time.

Remember to ease yourself into any of these activities slowly; this is your warm-up period. As you get warmer you can go faster, according to how you feel. At the end of the workout, taper off the speed, until you have slowed right down. Then record what you have done.

If possible, practise a variety of activities to develop your stamina. Go out for a walk/run once or twice a week, go for a swim, and go dancing as well. However, try not to do each activity to infrequently, as even though all these activities improve stamina (working on your heart and lungs), the muscles that the heart and lungs have to service are worked in different ways. If you leave too long a gap between periods of any one activity, you will suffer a certain amount of stiffness and soreness when you do get round to it again.

5

Strength: Weight Training

This chapter includes training methods to develop maximum strength, strength-endurance, and power, according to the various mixes of force, duration and speed.

As we saw in Chapter 4, *endurance* is generally regarded as the main component of 'fitness'. *Strength* is a lesser component, and plays its role in the concept of total fitness for the occasional moments when great force is required. For example, strength may be needed to change a flat tyre, carry heavy packages, dig the garden, force open a stiff window, and so on. The extremely 'fit' runner may have very durable legs, not necessarily very strong ones, but have little in the way of upper body strength. He can run to catch a train but may not be able to open a stiff window. A look at marathon runners shows that they often have very thin arms.

On the 'cosmetic' side of fitness, a reasonably symmetrical and muscled body may be desired, and this can only be gained by muscle-building work. A feeling of strength is an essential part of the business of feeling fit. When the muscles are regularly worked to the limits, there is often a resulting undefinable feeling of compactness, springiness, and all-round well-being. It feels good to be strong.

Many people prefer to exercise in a gymnasium rather than jog or join an exercise class. This chapter explains how both strength and stamina can be achieved using gym equipment and weights.

The various aspects of strength are achieved in different ways. Maximum strength is increased by working the muscles at about 80 to 90 per cent of maximum. Strength-endurance is developed by repetitive work against resistance outside the force-duration profile (see page 18) or above twenty-five repetitions. It can be achieved by raising maximum strength or, most commonly, by increasing the repetitions at the desired weight.

Power is increased by raising maximum strength and moving weights of above 60 per cent of maximum, as fast as possible. This power aspect of strength, however, does not affect the average person in quest of fitness, but athletes who have to define their sport very narrowly may need to work on it.

Strength is built up by gradually increasing the resistance against which the muscles have to work. This is generally done in two ways, using either the weight of the body alone or an external weight or piece of resistance equipment. The weight of the body can be used in many different ways depending upon whether maximum strength or strength-endurance is being developed. If all the bodyweight can be concentrated on one small muscle group it may be capable of only a few movements, for example, one arm press-ups or one legged knee bends. This would develop maximum strength in that muscle group. On the other hand, in press-ups the bodyweight is only partially on the arms and more than twenty-five repetitions may be possible, in which case strength-endurance is tested and worked upon.

The ability to use bodyweight alone to build up strength also depends upon age and sex. Whereas a young adult male would find bodyweight alone insufficient for maximum-strength training, an older or much younger person or female might well find bodyweight enough. A young adult male might also find that bodyweight alone was insufficient for strength-endurance work as he could build up to several hundred press-ups, for example, but would always be working against the same resistance. If he wanted to build up against a higher resistance he would have to use an external weight.

This chapter may therefore be of most interest to men, since the strength training methods described involve the use of weights. Although increasing numbers of women are becoming body-builders, the majority will probably get as much strength as they need from callisthenics or yoga (see Chapters 6 and 7). For those who do need to build up real strength, and not just body-tone, weight training is very suitable.

Many women fear that exercise will create large muscles. Although *any* exercise stimulates growth in muscle fibre, women do not respond in exactly the same way as men. The dominant hormone of the male sex hormones, testosterone, is responsible for gains in muscle size in men. Growth in muscle size is associated with lifting heavy weights, as when men lift heavy loads there is an increase in testosterone secreted. However, significant increases have not been found in women lifting heavy loads.

Whatever muscle growth is stimulated it is usually masked by the thicker layers of fat beneath the skin that women have, so the contours stay the same. Slight gains in weight due to muscle fibre increase are more than offset by fat loss, and the tape measure will actually show a decrease in size, as fat is bulkier than muscle. As with all forms of fitness training, those starting weight training or joining a gym are advised to undergo a thorough physical examination to determine cardiac, abdominal or any other weaknesses.

Using weights

Weight training is the main form of developing strength using an external load. It is mostly done using a barbell or dumb-bells, so the weight can be increased or decreased by adding or removing the iron discs at each end.

The advantage of this, and other types of weight-training equipment, is that the increase in weight can be accurately measured, and so a gradually increasing resistance can be applied to the muscles. The principle of weight training is *progressive overload*. That is, the muscles are progressively given more and more work to do. This is achieved by working to a formula of *sets* times *repetitions maximum* (RM). For many years the standard formula has been three sets of ten repetitions. A weight is moved ten times in a particular exercise. Then a brief rest is taken and the exercise is repeated. A final rest is taken, and the exercise is repeated for the last ten times.

There are two points that must be understood with the sets × RM formula with regard to increasing strength. Firstly it is a target. When you can do three sets of ten repetitions (or whatever number of repetitions you have selected), you have reached your target, and it is then time to increase the weight. Usually about a 5 per cent increase is made. For a while after you have increased the weight, you will not be able to achieve the number of movements. In the first set you may achieve ten movements, in the second set you may only be able to do eight, and in the final set you may only be able to do six movements. Over the following weeks you must keep working to achieve three sets of ten repetitions. When you do, you have made an increase in strength and it is time to increase the load by another 5 per cent or so (see page 51 for how to work out a routine).

The second point about the formula is that the weight used is the maximum. If you pick up a bar and move it ten times in three sets, but are in fact capable of moving it for three sets of fifteen repetitions, then you would not have been working at ten repetitions maximum. This refers to the maximum amount of weight you can move for the given number of repetitions. An exercise would progress with the first set comfortably performed, but with a slight feeling of 'burn' in the muscles. The second set would be done with probably a bit of struggle in the last two repetitions. The third set would be done with considerable struggle in the last four repetitions and a lot of 'burn' in the muscles. It is the number of repetitions you set yourself that determines the weight used. A period of experimentation is necessary at the start of any weight-training programme to find what weight you can move.

Within the sets × reps formula considerable variations are found. Sets or repetitions may be higher or lower and the weight on the barbell may be decreased or increased during the sets. Despite all the variations (and confusion), recent research seems to show that the greatest gains in strength are made with a formula of about three sets of about six repetitions with the same load on the barbell, and sufficient rest between sets.

When an increase in maximum strength is not the training objective, the sets × repetitions formula will differ. You may want to use the weights for a general workout – in other words to get the muscles toned-up, and have a sweat and a puff. Light to medium weights with high repetitions and sets, with not too much rest between the sets, will start to turn the session into an *aerobic* workout. This type of workout can be quite strenuous, as resistance may be quite high, compared with just moving the bodyweight as in running, and also may be prolonged (as with such sports as judo and wrestling). Pulse rates are pushed very high and trainees may develop extremely strong hearts despite the fact that there is a lot of anaerobic work going on (see page 14). This level of training would have to be achieved gradually.

If, on the other hand, you already do stamina work such as running, you may only need the weights to balance up your body strength. In this case the training could be done to a formula of three sets of ten repetitions with plenty of rest in between the sets.

If the training objective is to develop strength-endurance, then sets, reps, weights, and periods of rest will reflect the amount and type of endurance desired. There is no set point at which you acquire strength-endurance. Three or four sets of 15 to 25 RM with little rest in between may be all that is required. Alternatively, the trainee may just need to move a given weight many times continuously. He would then do a single set, gradually pushing the repetitions up to the desired number.

One of the advantages of training in sets is that between the sets the muscles have time to recover and replenish their energy stores. So, in a sense, the use of sets trains *recovery* as well. A quicker recovery would be gained by training with quite short intervals of rest between the sets.

Finally, your objective may be to build up your body, and to put on more muscle. Training advice to body-builders varies considerably. Some body-builders use very heavy weight at low repetitions, while others do many sets and higher repetitions. A lot depends on the individual body, as some will respond quickly to almost anything, and others will not respond without a lot of effort. However, one thing is very clear – all the methods advocated by the champion body-builders require an enormous amount of work. If you do a lot of exercises, and 'pump a lot of iron' in whatever formula, your muscles will respond.

The particular exercises for 'sculpting' the body for body-building competition are not included in this section, although any of the exercises will build you up considerably if enough work is done.

Equipment

A variety of equipment is now available for strength training in its various forms. The weights may be attached to pulleys, or fixed in a rigid frame and moved by leverage (i.e. multigyms). Weights may not be used at all, as with steel springs or rubber cables and pneumatic valve equipment. There are advantages and disadvantages with all this equipment.

Fixed frame apparatus is extremely convenient. The weight that is moved can be increased just by moving a pin. In contrast to this, free weights such as *barbells* and *dumb-bells* can be very fiddly when increasing or decreasing the weight and manoeuvring the equipment into position for the exercise. With the free weights however, the path of the movement is not fixed, as with the fixed frame equipment, and more muscles are called into play.

Equipment where work is against a *pneumatic valve*, or similar resistance-varying devices, is said to be the best for producing strength. The muscles have to work fully throughout the whole movement as compared to working with free weights, where a lot of effort is at the beginning of the movement, when the weight is jerked into motion. This type of equipment and movement is usually known as *isokinetic*. When using isokinetic equipment, the best strength gains are made by doing only one set of about fifteen repetitions, taking about four seconds to make the full movement. The results of this are about the same as doing three sets of five repetitions with weights.

Steel springs or rubber cables when used in such items as 'chest expanders' are very useful. There are a large number of upper body exercises that are easily done with the chest expander which are difficult to do with the free weights. However, the chest expander is not very good for leg, stomach, or lower back work.

In addition to the above, a gymnasium may contain a variety of machines for working different parts of the body, either moving the weight by pulley, leverage or isokinetically.

Technique

Always warm up before you go into your weight-training routine proper. If you train in a gym, use an exercise bike for about five minutes. Another useful warming-up exercise with a weight is the *dumb-bell swing*. Take a light dumb-bell in one hand, drop into a shallow squat and swing it between your legs. Straighten the legs, swinging the dumb-bell high over your head, then swing it down between the legs again, and so on. Do fifteen swings with one hand; then fifteen with the other. Go into a deeper squat as the exercise continues, and get a good stretch when it swings high. When pushing a heavy weight there is always the danger of tearing a muscle if you are stiff or not properly warmed up. One way to avoid this is to do a few yoga-type stretching exercises at the start and finish of a session. Also do a few light repetitions of any particular exercise before you load the bar properly.

Before using a bar or dumb-bell, check that there is the same amount of weight on each end of the bar, and that the collars that hold on the weights are firmly tightened. Hold the bar with your hands evenly spaced so that the weight is evenly balanced when you lift it. If using a bar regularly, mark off the exact middle and half-way to each side with a piece of tape.

When lifting a weight, lift with a flat back – never lift with a humped back. Also check that your feet and body are symmetrically placed. If using very heavy weights, get somebody to stand by to catch or support the bar, should you start to fall or fail in the exercise. When doing any exercise, concentrate on doing it in the correct form. Do not use weights that are too heavy and cheat on the movement. Try to work the muscles through their *full* range every time, and keep a record of what you do.

Routines

A general programme should consist of exercises for the arms and upper body, including chest, shoulders, and upper back; stomach; side; lower back, and legs. Reflecting the mobility of the various areas of the body, there will be proportionally more exercises for the arms and upper body than for the other areas. However, there is considerable overlap of the areas of the body that are worked with the various exercises.

Some of the following exercises are more exhausting than others. These are the ones where a lot of weight can be moved, such as the squat, bench press and dead lift, and also the composite power ones such as the clean and snatch. These should be spaced out in any one routine or done on different days so as to avoid complete exhaustion.

Those new to weight-training should start off with a *familiarisation* routine of one to three sets of about ten repetitions per exercise. The weight used should be light and the exercises few in number. At this stage the idea is to familiarise yourself with the exercise and its technique, and get the muscles accustomed to working in a new way against resistance. One way to start is to do one set of each exercise, then after a suitable rest move on to the next exercise and do one set, and so on through the routine. If, at the end of the list of exercises, you do not feel too tired, go through them again, and eventually, perhaps, a third time. After this point the routine is intensified by doing three sets of each exercise before moving on to the next one. This stage may take a few weeks.

The next stage of the routine is one of *consolidation*. At this point you have to start increasing the weight on the bar to find out your maximum for the stipulated repetitions. As before, work up to three sets of ten repetitions, slowly increasing the weight, and you will quickly discover your limits for that set-rep formula. Learning your limits should not take more than two or three weeks. From then on, providing that you train at least twice a week, you will find the strength work more and more comfortable. The maximum amount of weight you can handle should start to creep up, and your muscles will start to thicken. Aim for 5 per cent weight increases at a time.

At this point, when you have grown accustomed to the training, you can start to add a few more exercises, and experiment with the sets/reps/rest formula depending on your exact training objectives. When you have quite a few exercises for the arms and upper body in your routine, do not do them one after the other in sequence. Do one or two exercises for the area, then a stomach exercise, and then a leg exercise, moving down the body. Then go back and do the other arm and upper body exercises in the routine, and move on to any others lower down. This way you avoid totally exhausting one part of the body, to the detriment of the exercises for the other parts.

In general, stay with any routine you set yourself for about six to eight weeks. This will give you a chance to make some real progress, and then a switch to a slightly different routine will make a refreshing break. Switching to a new routine also helps to get over those sticking points when you do not seem to be able to get stronger. In some exercises you will make swift progress, others will prove more stubborn.

A typical routine might be:

Bench press
Bent-over rowing
Dumb-bell lateral raise
Biceps curl
Bent-arm pullover
Sit-ups
Back arches
Squat
Calf raise
Clean

This includes five arm and upper body exercises, two trunk, two leg and one composite exercise. Specialist weight trainers and body-builders often split their routines so that one day they concentrate on the upper body, and the next day on the lower body. However, this is when training several times a week with a lot of exercises for each part of the body.

Once into your training, do not lose sight of your overall fitness objective:

Stamina and muscle tone = Do 3 sets of 10 to 15 reps, medium to maximum weight, shortish rests, and a wide range of exercises.
Strength = Do 3 sets of about 6 reps maximum, with sufficient rest and as many exercises as you can manage.
Strength-endurance = Do 3 to 4 sets of 15 reps *over* 70 per cent of 1 rep maximum, or several sets of reps over 25. Little rest.

Power = As for strength *plus* moving weights over 60 per cent of maximum as fast as possible, rest as required.
Body-building = A lot of work in whatever formula, total poundage moved (multiply sets by reps by weight, and total up all the exercises) should be higher than most other types of routine.

When training for all-round strength, it helps to think in terms of movement rather than development of individual muscles. If you move a limb, it is easy to see or feel which muscles are called into play. However, the limbs move in a variety of directions, so it is necessary to work the muscles of the limbs in pushing, pulling and twisting movements. In this way the physique is strengthened in a well-balanced way.

The following weight-training exercises have been divided into pushing, pulling, straight, curl and twisting arm movements; trunk movements; extension, flexion, curl and straight leg movements, composite power movements and miscellaneous exercises for the neck, hands and feet.

Some of the possible body movements do not have an appropriate weight-training exercise because of the difficulty of devising one. There are very few arm-twisting exercises, for example. No doubt strength equipment manufacturers will eventually devise machinery for them. Physiotherapists and advanced body-building gyms do have many unusual pieces of equipment for these neglected movements.

Limb and trunk exercises

Arm pushing exercises

The hands can move out from the shoulders in a pushing action at many angles. When the arms extend in this way, the muscles at the back of the arms (triceps) are brought strongly into play and, depending upon the angle, the various muscles of the chest and shoulder girdle are involved.

5.1 Standing press The exercise starts with the weight supported at chest height, wrists and elbows under the bar. From this position the weight is pressed overhead to a full arm extension, then lowered to the chest again. As the weight is pushed up, the trainee looks straight ahead. When pushing a heavy weight, care should be taken that the stomach is not pushed forward with a lot of stress thrown on the lower spine. For such occasions, a wide leather training belt fixed tightly round the waist acts as a good support. There are a

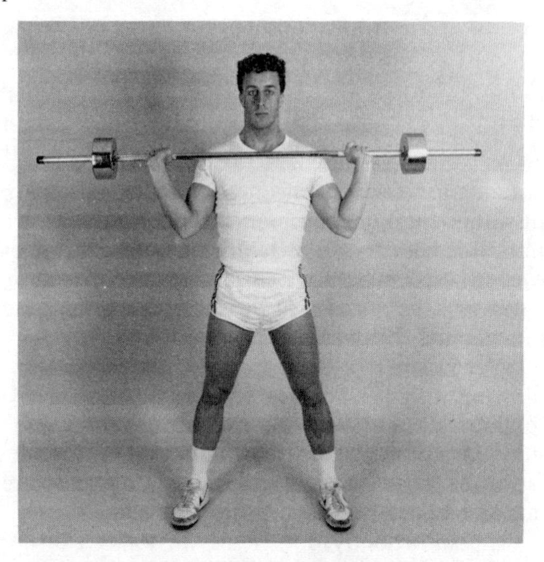

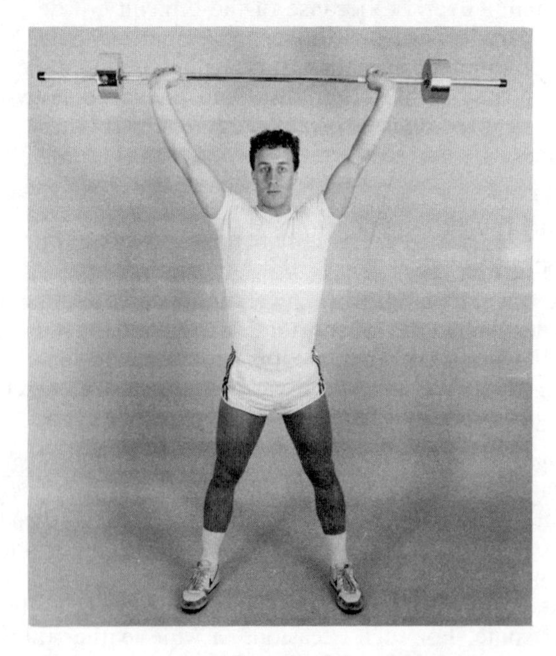

Exercise 5.1

number of variations on this exercise. A similar one is the press behind the neck.

5.2 Press behind neck In this exercise the starting position is with the bar held high, and it is then lowered behind the head to touch the nape of the neck, then pushed overhead again. The grip must be fairly wide, and the wrists and elbows should stay below the bar, as in the previous exercise. Both exercises can be done seated which throws some stress on the stomach as well.

Dumb-bells can also be used for the overhead pressing movements, in which case they can be pushed up together or alternately, with the hands either held palm forwards or facing each other.

5.3 Bench press In this exercise the trainee lies flat on a bench. The weight is pushed up from the chest till the arms are straight, then lowered, taking care not to bounce it off the ribs. When doing the exercise take care not to change the angle of the body, as there is a tendency when pushing a heavy weight for the hips to rise off the bench. Keep your back pressed flat to the bench, or do the exercise with both legs lifted and folded so that the thighs are vertical. The grip on the bar can be shoulder width or much wider. The change of grip affects the muscles in a slightly different way. The muscles affected are chest (pectorals), front deltoids and the triceps.

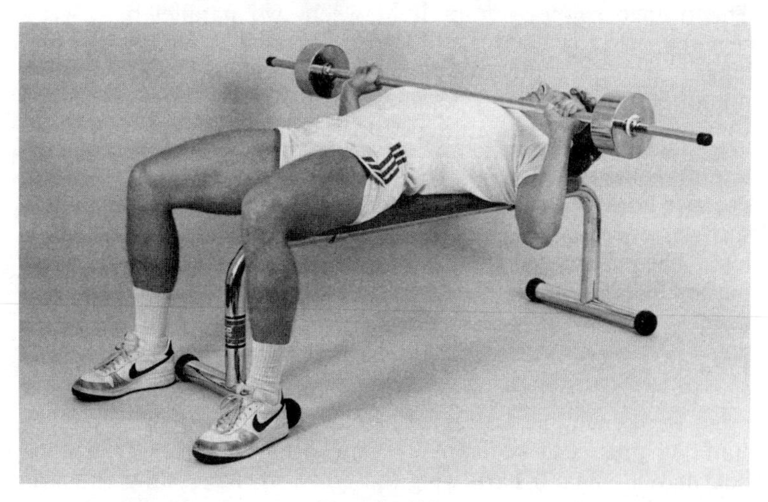

Exercise 5.3a

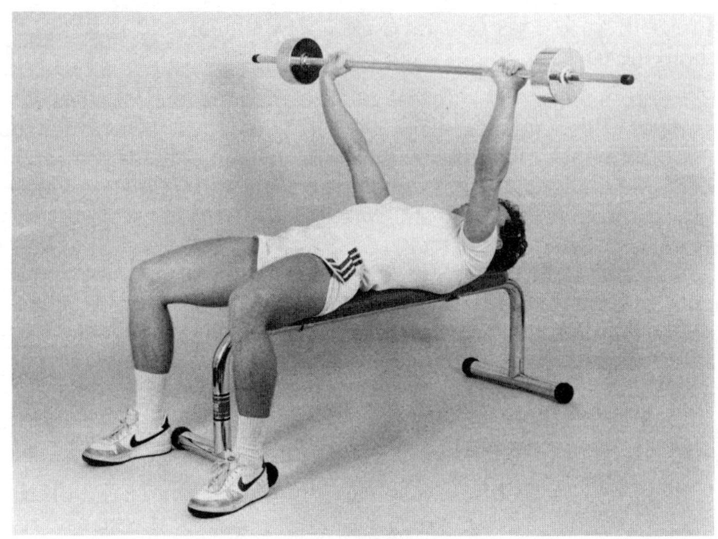

Exercise 5.3b

5.4 Dumb-bell bench press The previous exercise can also be done with dumb-bells, with the hands in the same position as with the barbell, or turned forward.

5.5 Dips This is an exercise that extends the arms downwards. The trainee supports himself between two parallel bars, arms straight, then lowers himself as far as the arms allow, then pushes himself up. Since this exercise uses bodyweight alone, and high repetitions are eventually possible, it later becomes necessary to tie some discs round the waist to overload.

5.6 Sideways extension The best piece of equipment for this exercise is the chest expander. Rubber cables are preferable to steel springs, since they do not catch the hairs on the chest or interlock. The expander is held across the chest or back, and the arms pushed directly out to the side. This is excellent for shoulder girdle development.

Variations Most of the arm extension exercises can be varied by slightly changing the angle of the body. For example, with the bench press the bench can be raised at one end or the other, and the standing press can be done by lying back on a steeply-inclined board. Widening or narrowing the grip also changes the effect on the muscles slightly.

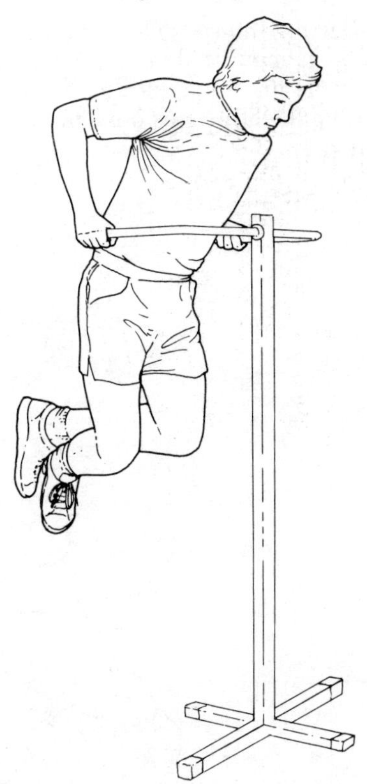

Exercise 5.5

Arm pulling (flexion) exercises
As with the extension exercises, the arm can be moved in to the body at many different angles. In these exercises, the muscles at the front of the upper arm (biceps) are strongly affected, as well as the muscles of the upper back and shoulders.

5.7 *Pull-ups* The trainee hangs from a bar, then pulls himself up to it. This can be done in a number of ways. Firstly, he can pull himself up so that his chin or chest touches the bar, or, secondly, touches the back of his neck to the bar. The grip can be either with both hands facing away from or towards the trainee, or alternated, with one forward and one backward. Depending upon which handgrip is taken, the grip can be wide, shoulderwidth, or narrow. This is a strenuous exercise and most people will find bodyweight more than enough. The very strong can overload by tying discs to the waist.

5.8 Lat pull-down This exercise has a similar effect on the muscles. It may be done on a separate overhead pulley or on a fixed-frame machine, and the bar is pulled down to the shoulders exercising the lattisimus dorsi muscle from which the exercise gets its name.

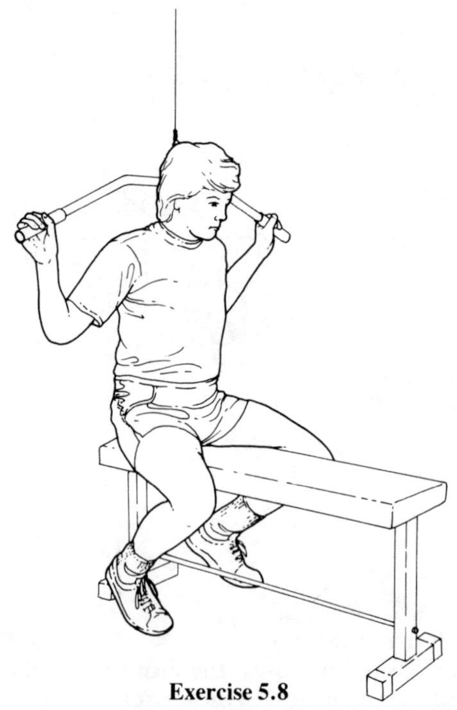

Exercise 5.8

5.9 Bent-over rowing This is the opposite exercise to the bench press. The trainee bends forward from the waist, preferably resting his head on something about waist height. The barbell hangs down at arms' length and is then pulled up to touch the chest. The hands should grip the bar about shoulder-width apart. When doing the exercise take care not to cheat by jerking the head and upper body up, as this then involves the lower back. Resting the head on something is a good way to avoid such cheating. The exercise can also be done with dumb-bells, with the hands turned in various positions. Some exercise machines have low-level pulleys, where the trainee sits on the floor and pulls towards his chest. This has virtually the same effect as the bent-over rowing.

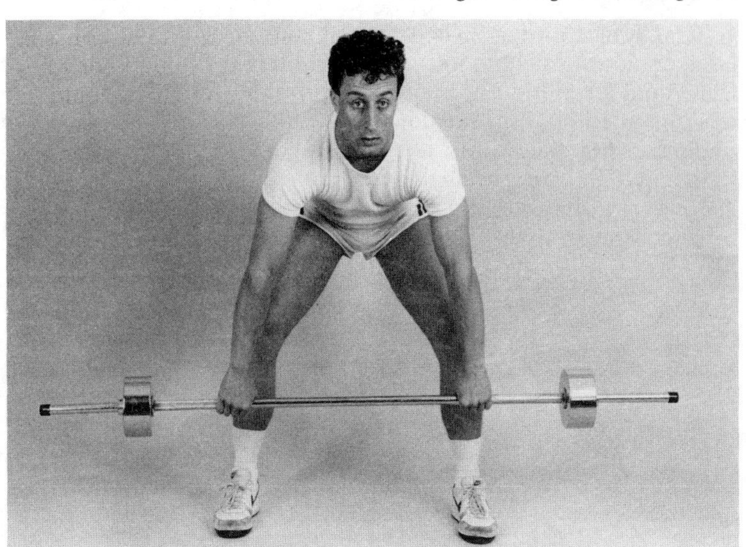

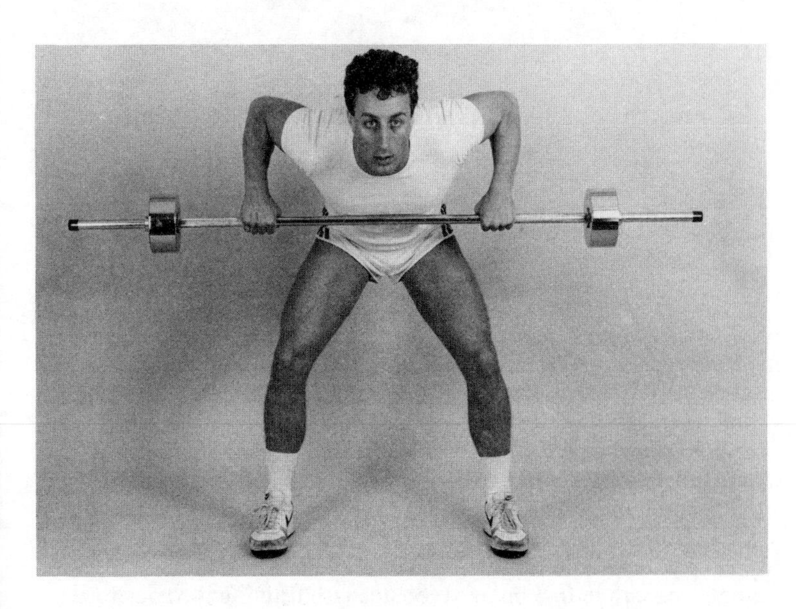

Exercise 5.9

5.10 Upright rowing The trainee stands upright holding the bar hanging at arms' length in front of the body, with a grip narrower than shoulder width. The bar is pulled up along the front of the body to stop under the chin, and down again. When the bar is brought up under the chin, the elbows should be higher than the bar, sticking up in the air. This exercise can also be done on low pulleys. A similar exercise is with two dumb-bells hanging at the side, and then lifted up under the armpits.

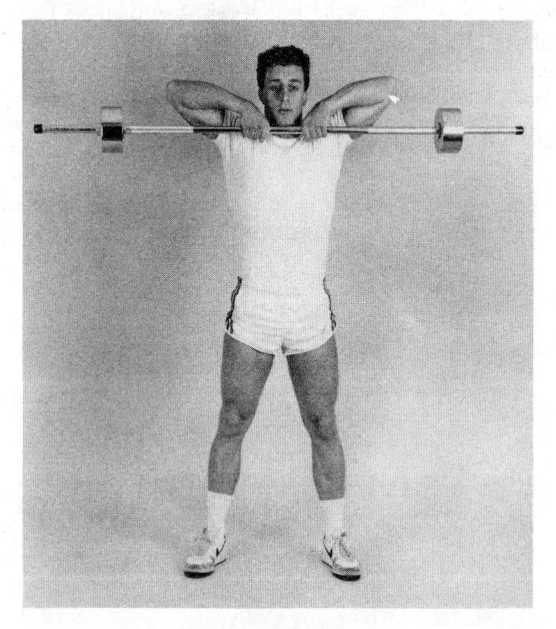

Exercise 5.10

Variations As with the pushing exercises, slight variations can be devised by lying or standing at different angles, and changing the grip or the spacing.

Arm twisting exercises

If you think of the action of using a screwdriver, you may recall how quickly the arm tires in the motion. No equipment exists for this type of exercise. Wringing out a wet cloth is a very similar movement, and can in fact be used for strength training if so desired. Do not forget to practise wringing out the cloth in both directions.

Straight arm exercises
When the arm is not bent and is lifted out and up, all the weight is thrown on to the shoulder muscles, particularly the deltoids. The muscles of the arm merely lock tight. Dumb-bells or chest expanders are ideal for this sort of exercise.

5.11 Dumb-bell lateral raise The dumb-bells are held hanging down by the sides and are then lifted up sideways, either to go just higher than the shoulders or right the way up to touch at the top. In the second case, the palms must be turned in to face each other when about shoulder height to make the full movement. A similar move can be made with the chest expander held in behind or in front of the body.

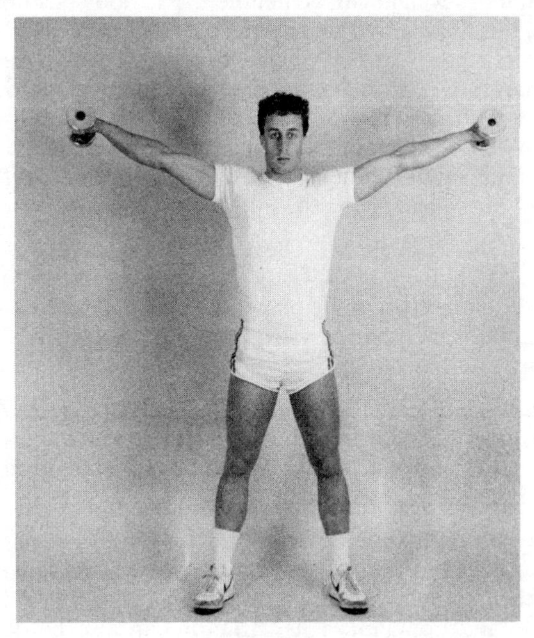

Exercise 5.11

5.12 Expander lateral pull-down This is the reverse movement to the previous exercise. The expander is held above the head, and the arms pull down straight and out wide to the sides.

5.13 Dumb-bell front raise The dumb-bells are held hanging down at the side, and are then lifted up to the front, arms straight, then above the head. Care must be taken that the weight is not swung up with a rocking motion of the body. Do the exercise fairly slowly and keep it well under control.

5.14 Straight arm pull-over This is the reverse movement of the previous exercise. The trainee lies on a flat bench, or on an inclined board with the feet higher than the head, and the barbell is lifted with straight arms from behind the head right round to touch the stomach.

5.15 Bent arm pull-over In this variation, the arms are bent, so that much more weight can be handled. The body position is much the same, but the hands may grip the barbell much closer together. In this exercise the arms stay bent throughout the movement, and the weight is moved from behind the head, round close to the head, to touch the chest. This exercise combines well with a breathing exercise. When the weight is lowered behind the head the ribcage is lifted, and this should combine with a deep in-breath. As the weight is swung over the head, breathe out.

5.16 Expander side-pulls The expander is held out at arms' length straight in front of the body, and then the hands pull out and round to the side on the same plane. A similar exercise can be done with dumb-bells, bending forward from the waist, then lifting them out and up.

5.17 Dumb-bell bench side raise This is the reverse of the previous movement. The trainee lies on a bench with dumb-bells held above the body at arms' length. The dumb-bells are lowered down and out to the side, then up again.

5.18 Bent arm side raise A slightly more popular variation of the previous exercise is the bent arm side raise, when heavier dumb-bells may be handled. The arms stay bent, and the weight is lowered to the side and up again. This variation can also be done on an inclined bench with the feet higher than the head, or vice versa.

5.19 Dumb-bell rear lift The trainee bends forward from the waist with the dumb-bells hanging down at arms' length. The arms are then lifted back and up past the side of the body. This has a limited range of movement, and strongly affects the deltoid muscles at the rear.

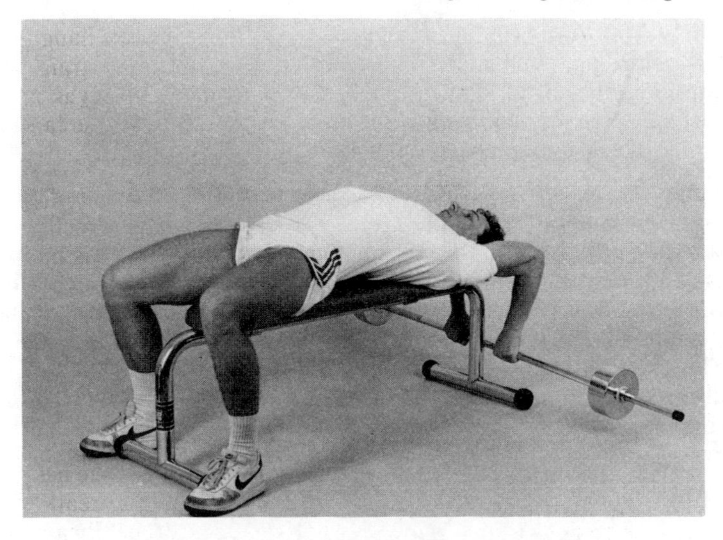

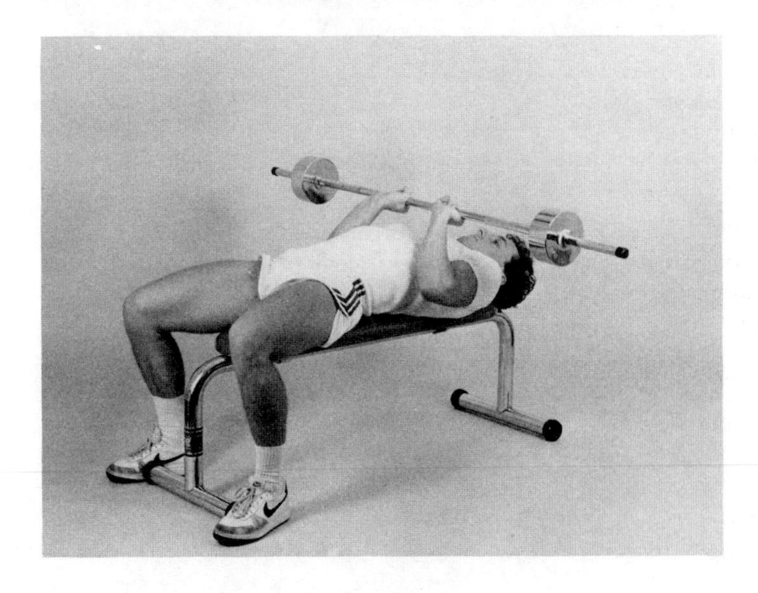

Exercise 5.15

Curls

All of the previous exercises work the arms and shoulder girdle considerably. However, by fixing the movement of the elbow, certain exercises can throw a lot more weight on to certain upper arm muscles, and so give them a more intense workout.

5.20 Biceps curl This is an exercise that can be done in many different ways. The simplest method is to use a barbell, when standing upright, with the bar hanging down at arms' length, palms facing forward, across the upper thigh. The bar is then 'curled' up with the elbows in a fixed position at the side of the body. By fixing the elbows, the muscles of the front upper arm take all the strain. This exercise can be done with dumb-bells with the hands turned in different positions – either knuckles forward, to the side, or to the rear. Each slight change of position affects different muscles in the arms.

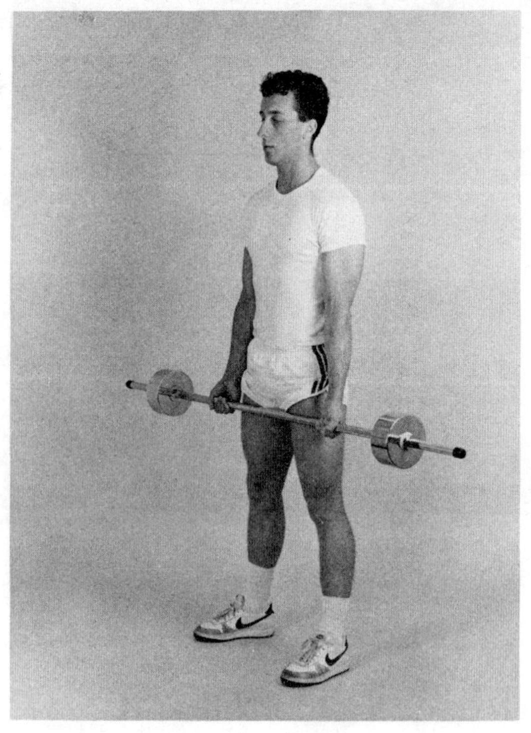

Exercise 5.20a

There is a tendency to 'cheat' in this exercise, as the body rocks back and forwards assisting the upward movement of the weight. When this is done deliberately, a lot more weight can be handled, and it is called a cheat curl. The upper arm can be immobilised in various ways to avoid any cheating. For example, the exercise can be done lying stomach down along a high bench with both arms hanging off the end, grasping the bar with the arms touching the supports of the bench. The weight is curled up as before, and the bench supports stop any movement of the elbows and upper arms. Body-building gyms have specialist benches for this sort of work.

When the exercise is done with a barbell held with knuckles forward, a lot more strain is thrown on to the forearms. This is sometimes known as the French curl.

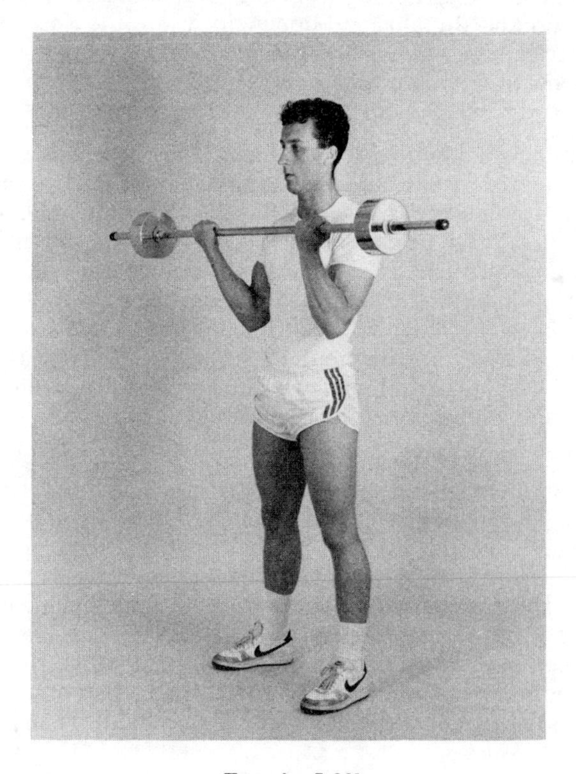

Exercise 5.20b

5.21 Triceps curl This exercise works the muscles at the back of the arm in the same manner as the previous exercise. There are not quite as many variations as with the biceps curl. A simple way to do the triceps curl is with a dumb-bell. Hold a single dumb-bell above the head, then keeping the elbow high and immobile, drop the dumb-bell down behind the head, then up again. A chest expander can also be used in various positions to work the triceps in a similar manner.

Trunk movements

If you sit in a chair and experiment with movement of the trunk from side to side, or front to back, you will see that it does not have a great range of movement. Of course it is possible to fold the body forward, or sway right back, but in these cases the trunk itself is not moving much, only folding from the hips, which means that the muscles around the hips and upper thighs are the ones affected. Weight-training exercises for the trunk usually involve folding movements from the hip area.

5.22 Sideways bend Stand with the feet nearly shoulder-width apart, holding a dumb-bell in one hand. The other hand can either hang at the side, or the hand can be placed at the back of the head. When doing this exercise, imagine that you are sandwiched between two sheets of fragile glass, so that no forward or backward movement is possible. The exercise is done by swaying to the side and letting the dumb-bell drop down the outside of the thigh, then swaying back the other way, and pulling the weight back up the thigh as high as it will go without bending the arm. The work is done when the weight is lifted, and it is the muscles of the trunk on the opposite side to the dumb-bell which are doing the work.

5.23 Side sit-up The muscles at the side of the trunk can be worked in a similar way in the side sit-up, which is a strenuous exercise. The trainee lies along a bench, but on his *side*, with the upper half of the body from the hips hanging off the end. So as not to over-balance, somebody must sit across the legs to hold them firmly in place. The exercise is done by clasping the hands behind the head and lowering the upper body towards the floor and up again.

Another way to work the muscles at the side of the trunk is to stand, feet about shoulder-width apart, with a barbell across the shoulders (check that the weights are securely held). Then just sway from side to side.

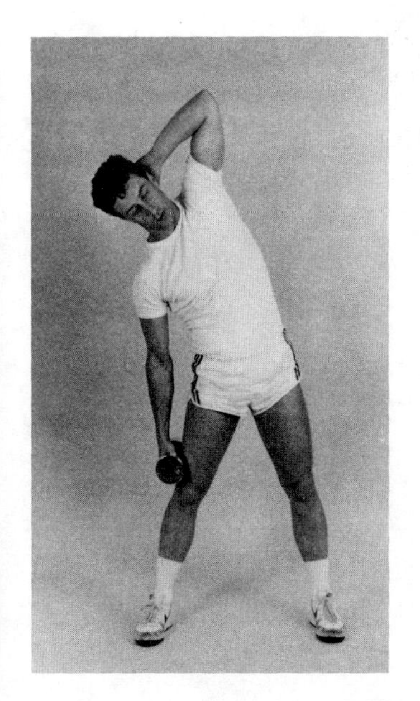

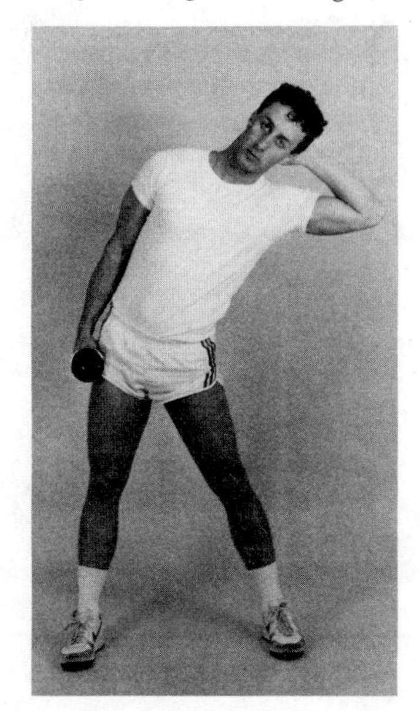

Exercise 5.22

Safety hint The following three exercises, back arch, good morning exercise and dead lift, are all very strenuous, and care should be taken that each exercise is first tried with very light weights, and that it is correctly done. Foot positioning and hand spacing on the bar must be symmetrical, and the movements must be done smoothly, in good form, and under control. Take care not to arch the back, but to keep it flat. Those with back problems should avoid these exercises altogether.

5.24 Back arch The muscles of the lower back are very strong, and so some of these lower back exercises can take a lot of weight (see Safety hint above). In this exercise the trainee lies stomach down on a bench, with the upper body down to the hips hanging off the end. The legs must be secured so as not to overbalance, usually by someone sitting on them. The hands are clasped behind the head, or kept at the side if that is too difficult, and the upper body is lowered to the floor and than raised as high as possible. When the upper body is lifted, the trainee must try to look at the ceiling, thus using muscles of the lower and upper back. This exercise is also known as hyperextensions or dorsal raises.

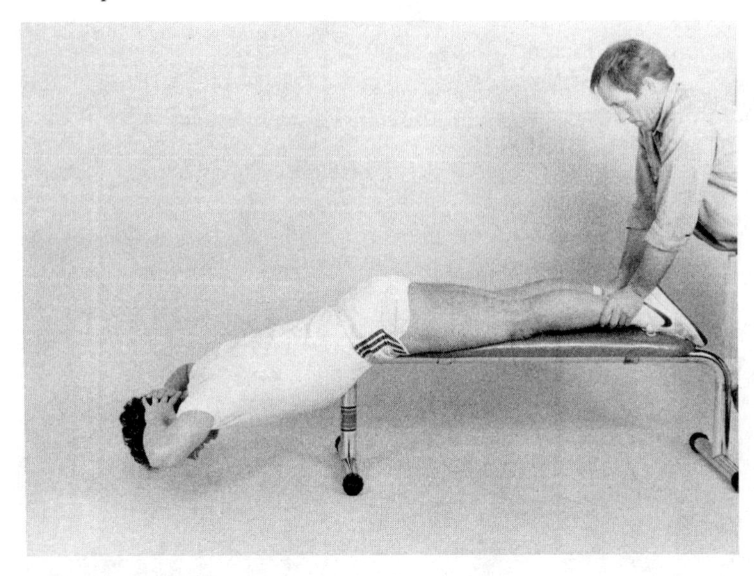

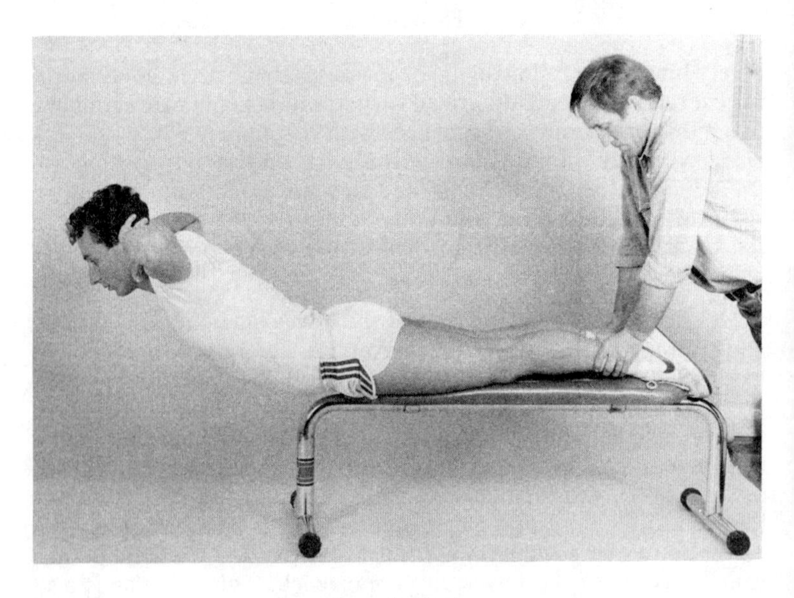

Exercise 5.24

5.25 Good morning exercise Stand with the feet about shoulder-width apart and hold a barbell across the shoulders. Keeping the legs straight and the back flat, bend forward from the waist till the trunk is nearly parallel with the floor, and then lift up.

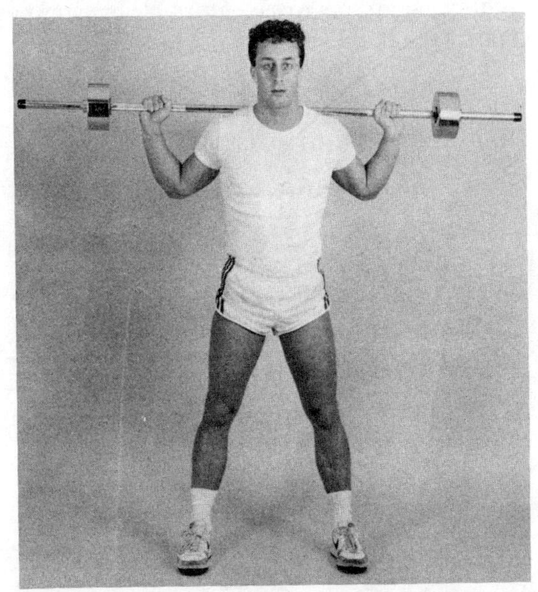

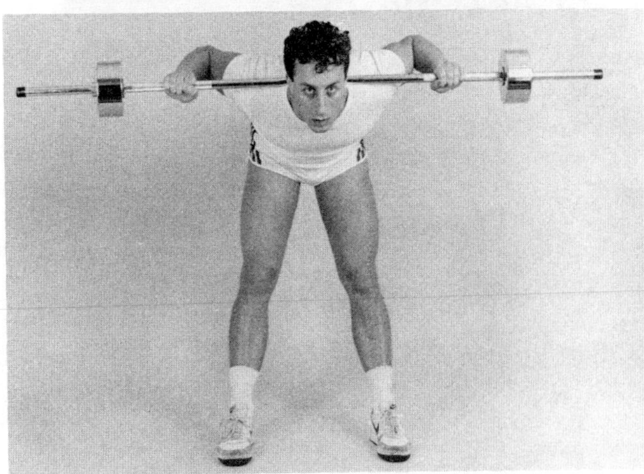

Exercise 5.25

5.26 Dead lift The barbell is placed on the floor. The trainee bends forward from the waist, keeping his legs straight, and lifts the bar up as high as it will go, without bending his arms or legs, so the bar will go no higher than the tops of the thighs. The weight is then lowered, not to the floor, but to a comfortable hanging position just above the floor, then raised again.

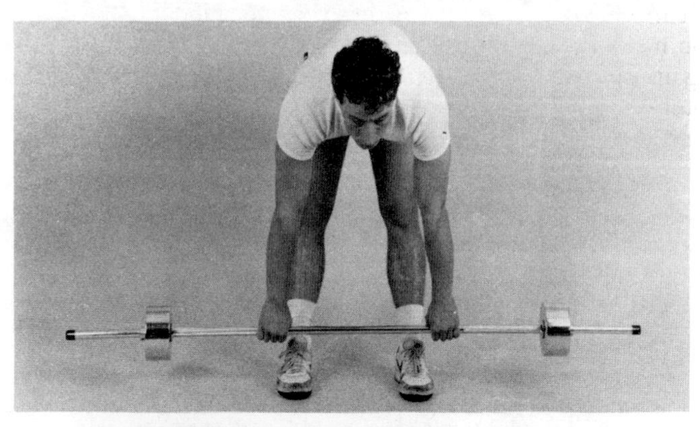

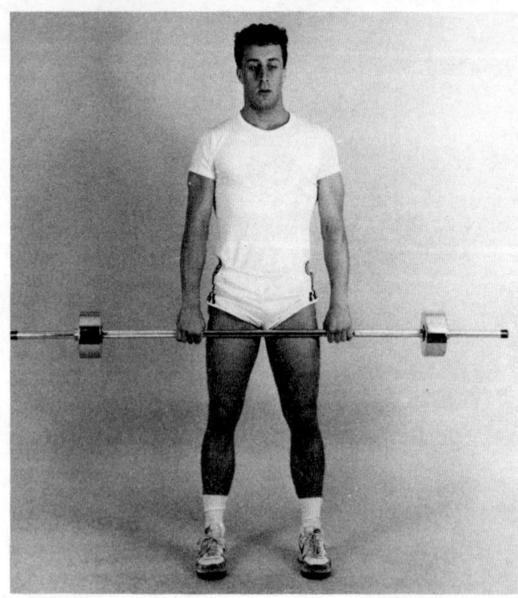

Exercise 5.26

5.27 Sit-ups In this exercise, as the name suggests, the trainee sits up from a supine position, thus working the muscles of the abdomen, hips and groin. There are many variations of this exercise. It is most easily done on a level surface, and can then be increased in severity by tilting the board or surface that is used so that the feet are much higher than the head. When the bodyweight alone can be easily moved, even on a very steep incline, the exercise can be made harder by holding a weight behind the head. When sitting up, bend the knees slightly. For other stomach exercises, see Chapter 6.

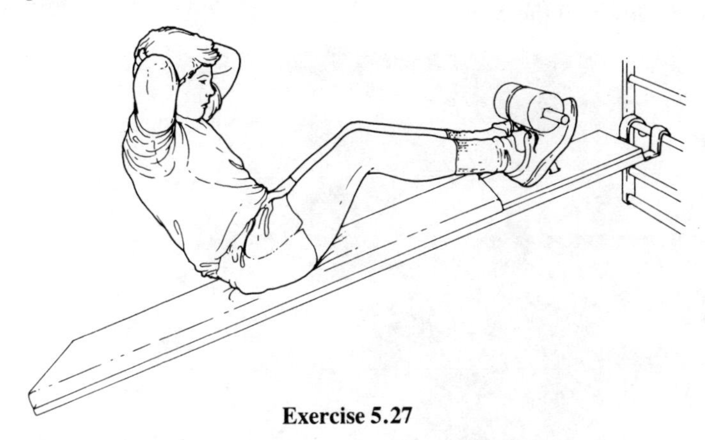

Exercise 5.27

5.28 Barbell swing This is an exercise that works the trunk in a twisting movement. The trainee stands holding the bar hanging down across his upper thighs, at arms' length. The exercise is done by twisting round to the left, raising the right-hand end of the bar as high as possible (check that the weight is securely fixed), then twisting the other way, raising the left-hand end of the bar, and so on. Push the stomach forward as you do the exercise and follow the bar with the head.

Leg exercises

The legs are not as dextrous as the arms, so have correspondingly fewer exercises. However, they are much stronger than the arms, and can take a lot more weight. Some people find this daunting, and avoid leg work somewhat. However, the squat is often called the 'king of the weight-training exercises' and should never be missed out.

5.29 Squat In this exercise the barbell is held across the shoulders, and the trainee squats, that is, he drops his buttocks and body close to the floor, then straightens up again. Sometimes it is necessary to put a block under the heels to make the movement comfortable. When doing the exercise, take care to push the chest out and pull the head back. Since it is believed that a full squat, that is, squatting as low as possible, loosens the ligaments of the knee, it is not done very often. Usually the exercise is done to a point where the thighs are parallel with the floor. Putting a lowish bench behind and squatting down far enough to touch it lightly helps to prevent going down all the way.

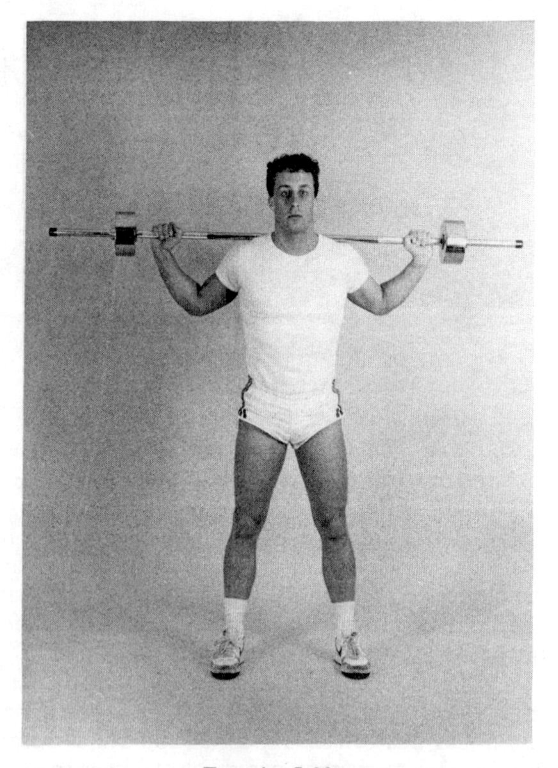

Exercise 5.29a

The squat can be done with the bar held in different positions, all of which affect the muscles of the leg in a slightly different way.

First, there is the front squat, where the bar is held resting across the upper chest, elbows locked under the bar. Then there is the Hack squat where the bar is held down behind the back, hanging at arms length across the buttocks. Blocks under the heels will be necessary for these exercises. The squat can also be of varying depths; the shallower the squat, the more weight can be handled.

Various machinery exists for the leg squatting movement. In the leg press machine the trainee lies on his back, feet up in the air, pushing up a weighted bar which slides up and down on two poles. When done this way, quite a lot of weight can be pushed up without the discomfort of supporting a bar across the shoulders as in the ordinary squat.

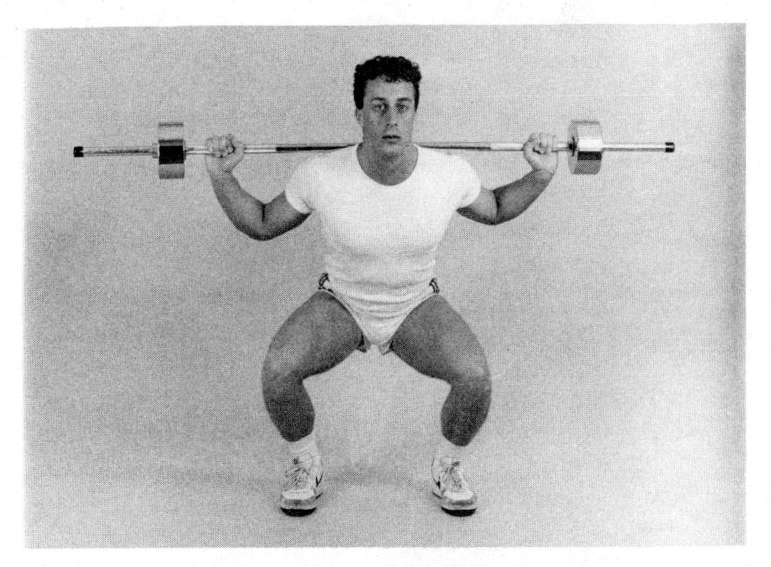

Exercise 5.29b

5.30 Calf raise The trainee stands with a weight across the shoulders and then rises on to the tips of the toes. To increase the range of movement, it is usually done with the toes on a block. The heels are then dropped as low as possible, then raised. Throughout the exercise the body and legs stay straight, so only the feet move to raise and lower the body and weight. Standard weight-training machinery exists for this exercise.

5.31 Leg extension This is the leg equivalent of the arm curls, as again, one portion of the limb is fixed, and the other moves against the extra resistance. Standard machinery exists for this movement, although it can be done without. The trainee sits on the leg extension machine and, holding the upper body and thigh still, pushes the pad against his ankles to maximum extension of the leg. This is an excellent exercise for weak knees (quadriceps), and is much used by footballers in training, or in recovering from knee injuries.

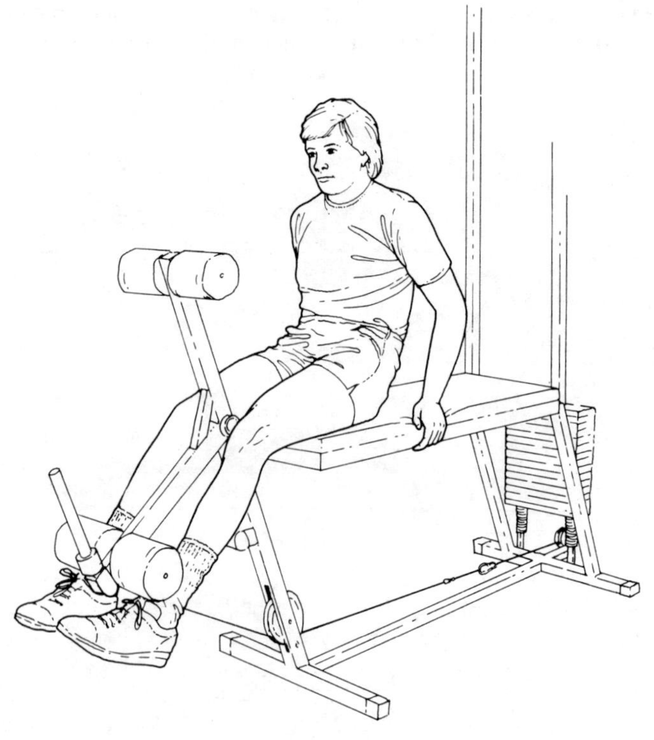

Exercise 5.31

5.32 Leg curl Here the curling action is the reverse of the previous one, so that it is the muscles at the back of the thigh which are worked. The trainee lies flat down on his stomach, and hooks his heels under the pad of the leg-curl machine. The pad is then curled back with the trainee pulling his feet round to his buttocks.

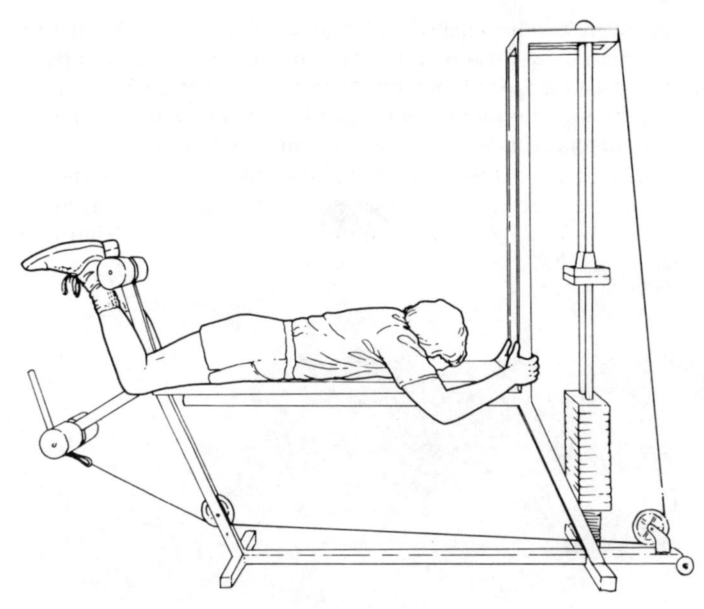

Exercise 5.32

5.33 Straight leg raises This is a fairly rare exercise in which the trainee wears an iron boot which also has an attachment for putting on extra weight. Standing straight on one leg, the other weighted leg is lifted directly sideways or forwards, with the leg kept straight throughout.

Composite power movements

There are few exercises in which the weight, barbell or dumb-bell, is lifted up to the chest or above the head in one heave. These exercises involve a number of muscle groups, which makes them quite strenuous. Since the whole body is used, a lot of weight can be lifted. However, heavy weight cannot be lifted slowly, and these movements are done explosively, combining strength with speed, and so demanding *power*. These are the sort of movements used in Olympic weight lifting.

5.34 Barbell clean to chest The trainee squats slightly, grasping the bar symmetrically. A deep breath is taken, then the bar is swiftly lifted up to the chest in a standing position, locking briefly in position with the elbows and forearms under the bar, then dropped to the floor, not to crash down, but to touch lightly before being lifted again. Care must be taken that the legs are bent to start with, that the back is kept flat and not humped, and that the legs, back and arms work together in one big explosion to blast the weight high. A similar exercise can be done with one or two dumb-bells.

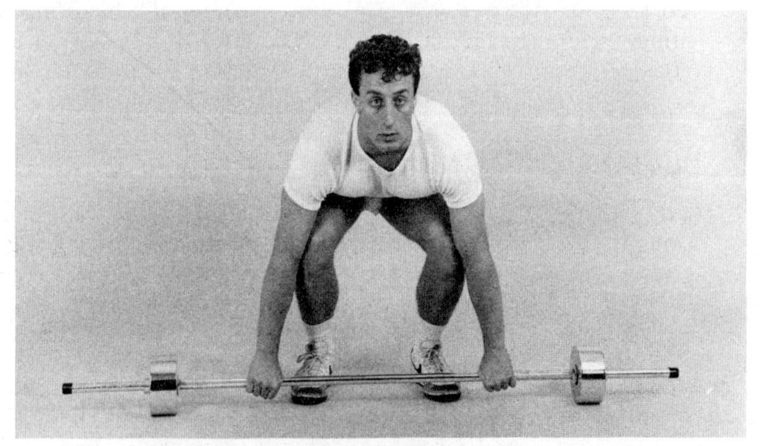

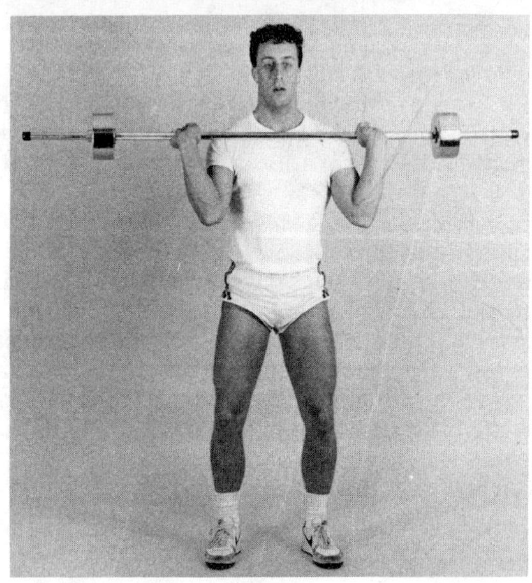

Exercise 5.34

5.35 Snatch above head In this exercise the weight is lifted in one smooth movement right above the head to a full outstretched arm position. The body can be dropped lower under the bar either by going into a deep squatting position or into a wide front to back lunge position. However the legs are placed, the weight must be lifted to a full outstretched arm position above the head in one continuous fast movement. Dumb-bells may also be used for this exercise.

Miscellaneous exercises

There are a number of exercises for the neck, hands, and feet, although these are mostly done without weights. A few strength exercises, done with weights, do exist, and these are described below:

Neck exercises

5.36 Wrestler's bridge The Wrestler's bridge is a very common way to work the neck, and can also be done using extra weight. The trainee lies down on his back on the floor, and draws his feet close in to his buttocks. Something soft (but securely placed to avoid sliding) must also be placed under the head. The exercise is done by bridging up – that is, by lifting the body right off the floor so that it is supported on the head and feet, and then lowering it again. When the neck is strong enough, the bridge can be done supporting a barbell above the body at arms length.

5.37 Head harness Another way to work the neck is with a head harness. This is a webbing device which fits over the head and has straps hanging down to which weight can be attached. The weight is then lifted by raising or moving the head.

The neck responds very quickly to exercise and can thicken considerably. This is worth bearing in mind when it comes to buying shirts – the collar may soon be too small!

Wrist exercises

The wrist itself does not have muscles to exercise, as it is a joint. Usually this heading refers to exercises that involve wrist movements, but which in fact work the muscles of the forearms.

5.38 Wrist-roller The wrist-roller is a simple and common piece of equipment. A short length of rope is fixed to the middle of a short round pole. A weight is attached to the other end of the rope and the weight is then wound up by rotating the pole. The arms stay fairly straight through the exercise with just the hands turning the pole, first one way, then the other.

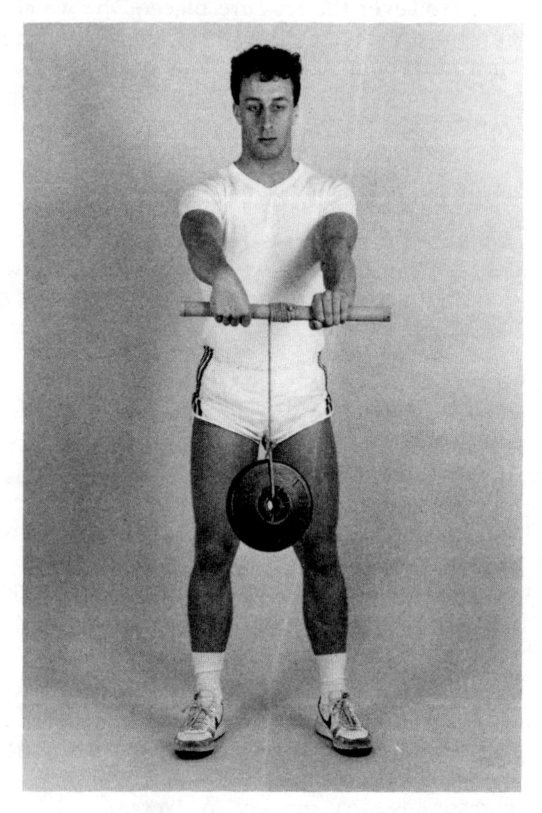

Exercise 5.38

5.39 Wrist curl Another exercise for the forearms is the wrist curl. In this exercise the trainee rests his forearms on a flat surface such as a bench, with his hands, palm upwards, hanging over the side holding a barbell. The exercise is done by lifting the weight as high as it will go, knuckles curling in towards the forearms, then lowering it, unclenching the hands so that the bar rolls down to be held by the last joint of the fingers. The fingers then pull in again, and the hands lift the bar, and so on. The forearms do not leave the flat surface at any point.

Points to remember

You must proceed carefully with weight training. Weights incorrectly moved can cause injury. As you train, each muscle group is exercised to near exhaustion and, if you are not used to it, the effects may suddenly accumulate to the point where you feel sick or are sick. Older people should never hold their breath and strain against high resistance.

As a general rule, it is best to get expert tuition and supervision in a gym, at least while you are new to weight training.

6

Callisthenics

Callisthenics are literally exercises which are suitable for producing strength and beauty. These exercises are free-standing ones where the weight of the body alone is used for resistance. They are the sort of exercises usually done in physical-training or keep-fit classes in a gymnasium but can equally well be done at home. Fitness-orientated dance movements also come into this category.

The results obtained from such exercises depend on how they are used. If stamina (circulo-respiratory endurance) is required, the work has to be fairly fast and continuous. Except for the very young or elderly, callisthenics are not much good for increasing maximum strength. All a young male would get out of them would be stamina and strength-endurance. However, callisthenics can be put together in a considerable variety of ways to include stretching and dance movements, to produce graceful, stylish routines.

A well thought-out, imaginative callisthenics class is probably one of the best ways of working out. All parts of the body can be worked on, and strength, endurance, suppleness and style are developed. Given a large, well-equipped gymnasium, competitive games can also be introduced to add to the fun.

The easiest way to do callisthenics is to join a class. The teacher then has to do all the work of putting together a balanced routine, and you only have to carry out instructions. At present, some of the best classes around are for women, and are mostly done to music with a bias toward dance movements. However, many men would find them very tough workouts and should try them. Since there are many variations on this theme, it is best to look around to find the type of workout that suits you best.

One of the advantages of callisthenics is that they can be done virtually anywhere. Whether you are at home or away, they can be done in any small space available, such as a bedroom. The only difficulty of doing callisthenics alone is sustaining interest, so join a class if you can. If you are exercising alone, try to use music with a good, strong beat, as this will keep you going. There are a number of exercise records and videos on the market, although some of the voice-overs can be irritating. The beat used for exercises varies, but it is not difficult to put together something yourself which includes your favourite music.

If you are using a callisthenics session to develop stamina, the work must be more or less continuous and fairly fast. In this case you cannot spend too much time on the *form* of the exercise, as a dancer would. The musical beat for the standing exercises should be quite fast. For the floor exercises use a slower beat if continuing to work on your stamina, or some slowish music, such as Tchaikovsky's ballet music, if concentrating on form.

You can increase the benefits you get from these exercises if you take care to do them properly, that is, making sure the lines of the body are straight, with legs straight and toes pointed, and so on.

If you merely go through the motions you will not benefit very much, so put some life into the movements. Where the exercise requires a good stretch, make sure that the movement into the stretch is slow and strong, and not a violent jerk. If you find that you cannot quite do the exercise because of stiffness, do not change the form of the exercise. Aim to achieve the required suppleness over a period of time by carefully working the stiff parts in the correct way.

The following exercises are grouped according to the starting position. The first sections cover the very active exercises done on the feet, then are followed by the slower ones done on the floor. If you are working out alone, try to remember the general progression of the positions. Once you remember a position and get into it, several exercises will come to mind. Most of the exercises are very straightforward; however, the more difficult ones are marked *strenuous*. The unfit or the elderly must avoid these.

Although many exercises are described, you will not find it difficult to remember them if you can remember the progression through the various starting positions. To summarise, these are:

Running on the spot
Hopping and leg raises
Jumping

- Standing
  - feet together
  - feet apart
- Crouching
- Kneeling
- Sitting
  - straight-legged
  - legs wide
  - cross-legged
  - Indian cross
- Lying
  - Back lying
  - Side lying
  - Front lying
- All-fours

The first three groups are good for stamina. They will raise your pulse rate and make you breathe hard. Much the same effect can be gained from the rest if you work at them hard and fast. However, you may wish to slow down somewhat to concentrate on form and good stretch.

A few of the exercises are *isolation* exercises. That is, they work on isolated muscles. A good example of this is the shoulder-rolling exercise. Most of the exercises work several parts of the body at the same time so that there is an overall toning up effect.

If working alone, some experimentation will be necessary to put together a session of the right length. Select three exercises each from the Running, Hopping and Jumping sections and do them for twenty repetitions each. Go through the nine exercises once or more until you feel that you have had a good puff (try checking your pulse rate). This should take a mimimum of five minutes. As you start to remember the exercises, you can add more from these sections, moving vigorously until you feel that you have done enough. If recording your own music, leave a few seconds gap between each track, and use it for breathing exercises or a short rest. The chart below shows an example of a basic workout, which should take about fifteen minutes. To extend the duration of the workout add more exercises per exercise group and/or increase the repetitions. To increase the intensity of the workout do the exercises faster with less rest in between and add more of the exercises marked *strenuous*. The first exercise can be used as a gentle warming up, in which case run softly on the spot for a few minutes then move into the rest of the routine when you feel warm and begin to puff.

Exercise	**Repetitions**	
Running on the spot		Repeat first three sections
6.1 Running on the spot	20	
6.3 Kicking the bottom	20	
6.8 Rope climb	20	
Hopping and leg raises		
6.13 Basic movement	20	
6.15 Front kicks	20	
6.17 Side leg raising	20	
Jumping		
6.20 Hip twists	20	
6.23 Astride jumps	20	
6.25 Lunge jumps	20	
Standing (feet together)		
6.27 Fountain	10	
6.28 Ski and stretch	10	
Standing (feet astride)		
6.37 Sky reach	10	
6.43 Side bends	10	
Crouching		
6.48 Squat twists	10	
6.49 Head to knee	10	
Kneeling		
6.51 Side swing	10	
6.52 Kowtow	10	
Sitting (straight-legged)		
6.55 Knee and toe touch	10	
6.56 Arm swing	10	
Sitting (legs wide)		
6.61 Seated twist	10	
6.62 Side bend	10	
Sitting (cross-legged)		
6.63 Elbow to knee	10	
6.64 Crawl	10	

Exercise		Repetitions
Sitting (Indian cross)		
6.67	Swirl	10
6.68	Reach and sway back	10
Lying (on the back)		
6.74	Leg swings	10
6.76	Heel kicks	10
Lying (on the side)		
6.78	Side leg raises	10
6.79	Knee to shoulder	10
Lying (on the front)		
6.82	Leg raises	10
6.89	Butterflies	10
All-fours		
6.90	Leg swings	10
6.96	Mule kick	10

After the first three groups, progress through the rest of the starting positions, taking two exercises from each, and doing ten repetitions. Where the exercise is a left to right movement, or is with one limb, count ten to the left and ten to the right. The number of exercises and repetitions can be increased as you get fitter.

Under the first three headings are the really active exercises that will give you a good stamina workout. A good fifteen minutes or more should be spent on these exercises. If you are not concentrating on stamina, you should finish with a minute or two of these exercises or interpose them at any time to liven up the pace. Apart from raising your pulse and making you breathe harder, the muscles of the legs are given a good workout.

Running on the spot

6.1 Running on the spot This can be from very slow to very fast, with knees lifted to different heights.

6.2 Toe stretch This has to be done in bare feet, and fairly slowly. Instead of lifting one foot off the ground each time, keep it in contact with the ground, but step right on the tip of the toes, then roll your foot forward and under, so that the big toe nail touches the floor.

6.3 Kicking the bottom Try to kick your bottom with your heels as you run on the spot.

6.4 Forward lean Lean forward as you run, and swing your arms across your body, as if toiling up a long steep slope.

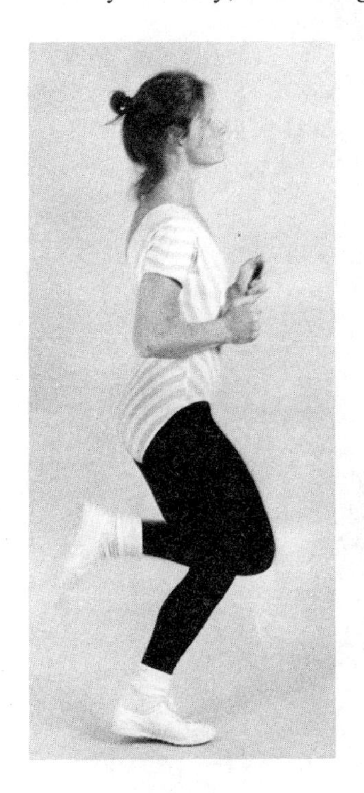

Exercise 6.3

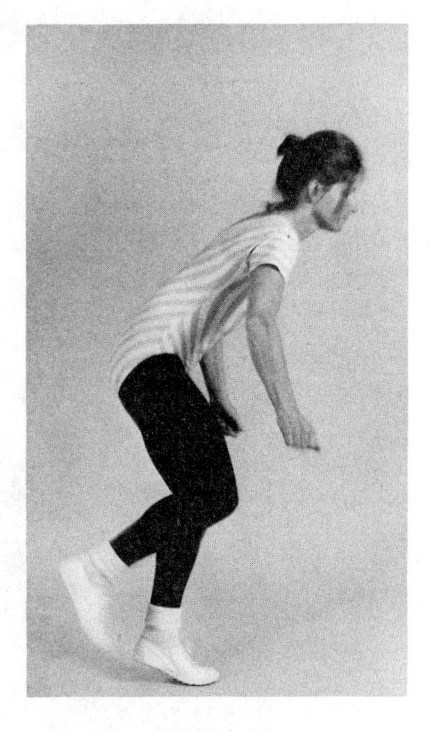

Exercise 6.4

6.5 Lean back Lean backwards as you run, lifting your knees high, and wave your hands at shoulder height in front of the body, as if in a chorus line.

6.6 Wave As you run, wave your arms from side to side above your head, as if acknowledging the cheers of a crowd.

6.7 Shoulder dip As you run, drop each shoulder in an exaggerated dip down to the side. To exaggerate the action further, point down to the floor with your index finger as you drop your shoulder. The hip movement can also be emphasised.

6.8 Rope climb As you run on the spot, reach up alternately with the arms, as if climbing a rope ladder. Alternatively, keep both arms high in the air, and edge each hand in turn an inch or two higher than the other.

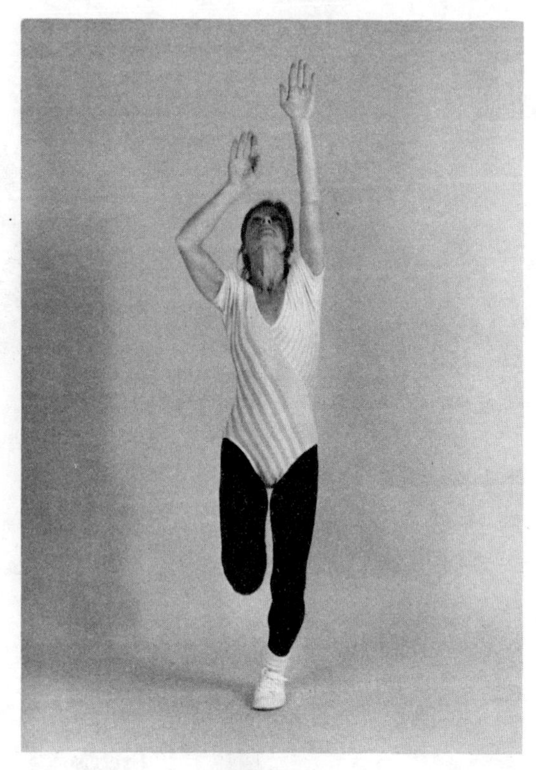

Exercise 6.8

6.9 Leg splay As you run, splay each foot out to the side and back. Also touch each foot with your hand.

6.10 Back cross Instead of splaying the leg out to the side, cross it behind the other leg. Also touch each foot with the opposite hand. You could exaggerate the action by lifting the foot so that the sole comes uppermost, and look at each sole.

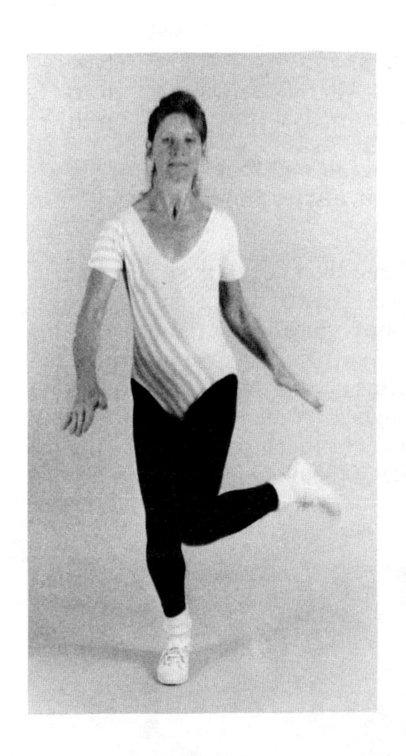

Exercise 6.9

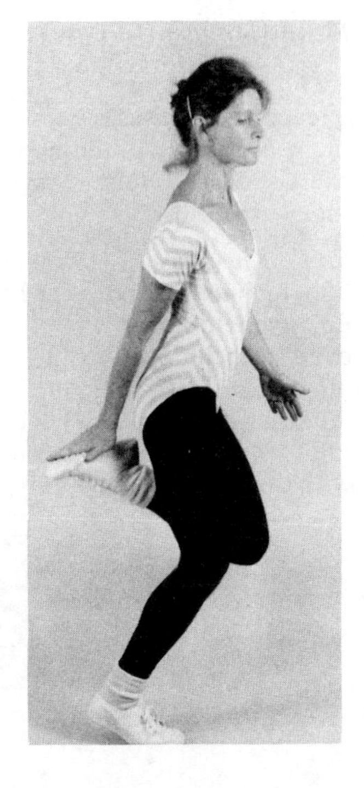

Exercise 6.10

6.11 Swerving Cross one leg in front of the other, and vice versa, in a continuous exaggerated swerving motion. Also exaggerate the twisting of the hips (but take care not to trip).

6.12 Interjections As you run, insert various arm movements, such as windmilling the arms either way, in small or large circles. Also clench the fists at the shoulder, and flick the arm up, down, out to the side or front, stretching out the fingers with the arm fully extended. You could also add an occasional scissor jump, with the legs making a quick imitation of a pair of scissors opening and shutting. Also try a star jump (*strenuous*). Drop into a crouch, fingers touching the floor, then leap up, spreading out arms and legs in a star shape.

Hopping and leg raises

6.13 Basic movement The basic movement for this next sequence of exercises is a single hop on one foot, then a single hop on the other foot. As the hop is made on one foot, the other leg is exercised in different ways. First of all just try hopping on each leg in time to the music.

6.14 Knee raise As you hop, bend the knee of the other leg and lift it high to the front. The lift can be assisted by the hands pulling it up, even to touch the upper body. Further variations on this exercise include lifting the knee and swinging it across in front of the other leg. As this is done, the arms should swing the other way. Alternatively, lift each knee out high and wide to the side, pointing the toes down. Another variation is to touch each knee as it rises with the elbow of the opposite side of the body.

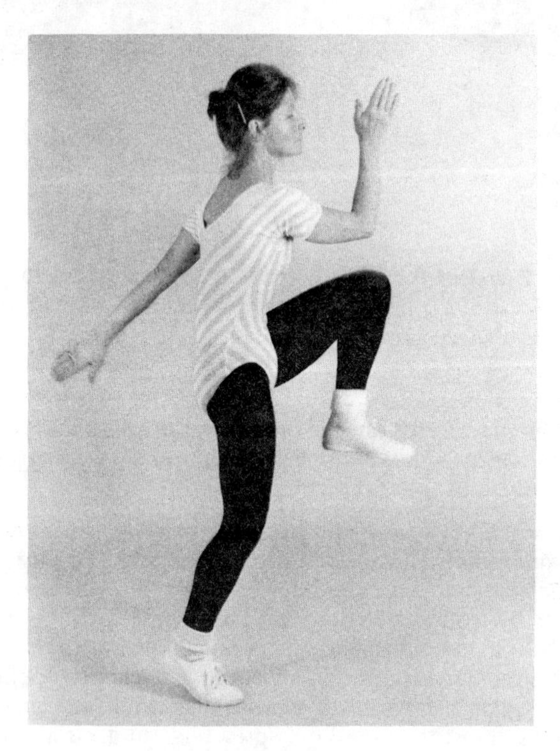

Exercise 6.14

6.15 Front kicks As the hop is made on one leg, the other leg kicks out to the front, karate style. (That is, the knee is lifted high, and then the foot flicks out.)

6.16 Straight leg raising As one leg hops, the other leg is lifted straight up to the front, in chorus-line style. The leg can be raised to waist height, or even up to face height if possible. The hands can be placed on the hips or extended out to the side, and the back should be straight. Variations include touching the foot as it comes up, with either hand, or clapping the hands under each leg as it rises.

6.17 Side leg raising Swing each leg high to the side with a hop on the supporting leg in between. The hands can either rest on the hips or be extended to touch the toes.

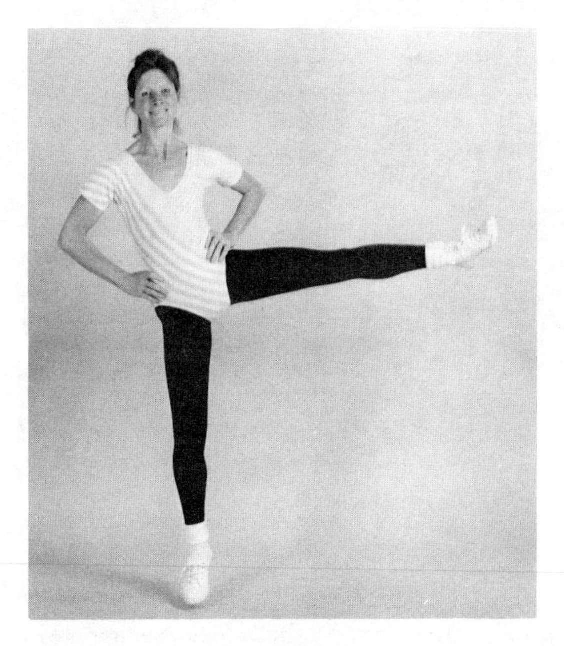

Exercise 6.17

6.18 Front and back leg raising Swing one leg up to the front, then bring it back to the ground, doing a hop on it as the other leg swings back and up. Hold the arms out straight to the side and lean forward as the leg swings back, and then straighten up as the other leg goes forward. You should change legs every few swings.

6.19 Flea-hop This exercise begins balancing on the right leg, leaning forward from the waist, with the left leg extended backward, slightly bent. Let either arm hang down to the ground. Then make one hop in to the centre, *jump* onto the other leg reversing all the body positions, and hop in to the centre again, and so on. The sequence is: hop in, jump onto the other leg, hop in, jump to the other leg.

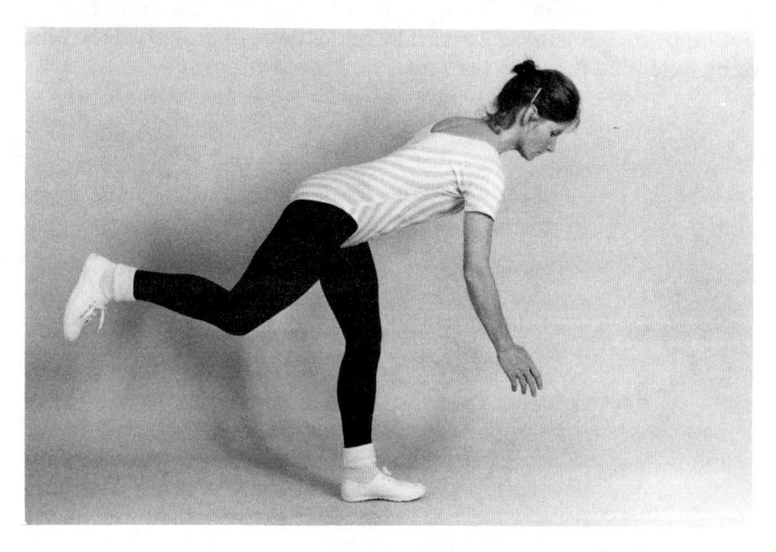

Exercise 6.19

Jumping

6.20 Hip twist Jumping with both feet together, twist the hips and legs to the right, then to the left, keeping the shoulders facing forward all the time. Variations include swinging both arms together in the opposite direction to the knees or holding both arms high above the head, fingers touching. An extra jump can be interposed at each turn to the side.

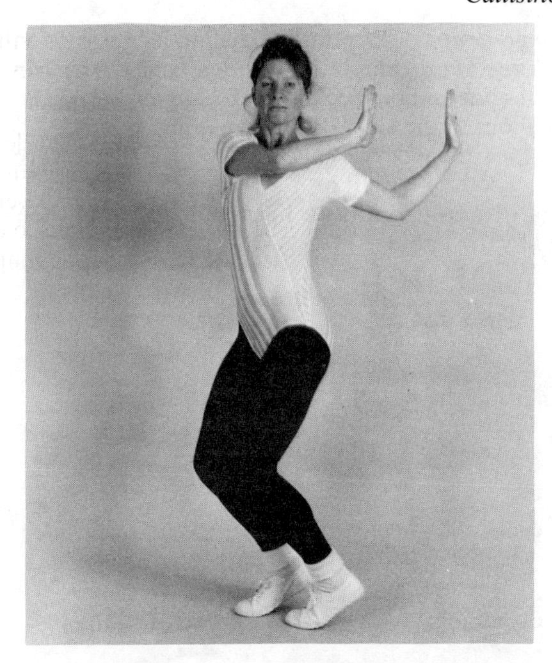

Exercise 6.20

6.21 V-jumps Jump out diagonally to the front with both feet together. Jump back to the starting position then jump diagonally out to the front the other side. Imagine you are jumping out along a large V-shape. Add to the exercise by opening your arms out high and wide to the side, from a crossed position on the chest, as if acknowledging the cheers of an audience.

6.22 Jumps into half-squats Jumping with feet together on the spot, leap forward into a half-squatting position and back again.

6.23 Astride jumps Jump with feet astride, then feet together, and so on. Also try the exercise with the arms moving straight out and up from the side, touching hands above the head as the feet land astride, and coming back down by the sides as the feet come together.

6.24 Side jumps Jump both feet together out to the side, leaning in towards the centre, and then over to the other side. At each landing point add an extra bounce.

6.25 Lunge jumps Drop into a fencing-lunge position (one leg forward, knee bent, other leg extended back). This can be done with an extra hop or bounce before exchanging leg positions. Arms can be held out to the side, or hands placed on hips. The arms can also swing forward and back (one each way), either left arm with left leg (and vice versa), or left arm with right leg and vice versa. This exercise is *strenuous* if a deep lunge is made, and should not be attempted by the unfit.

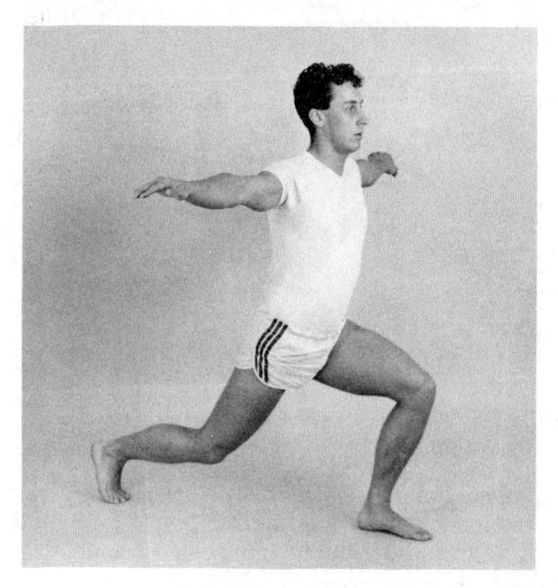

Exercise 6.25

6.26 Side leap Start with legs wide apart. Sway the shoulders right over to one side, so that the leg on the other side leaves the floor, and then make a small leap off the supporting foot. Then sway the shoulders over to the other side, and leap again. Take care to sway the shoulders over in an exaggerated manner, otherwise the exercise will turn into the hopping side leg raise.

Standing

This group is subdivided into standing with feet together and standing with feet astride.

Feet together

6.27 Fountain Stand with the feet together. Bend both knees into a deep crouch. As you do this, touch the floor in front of your toes with both hands and, as you straighten your legs, bring your hands up, palms together, in front of your body, and stretch up as high as you can above the head. As your hands go above your head, swing your arms wide in a large circle back down to the floor, bending your knees again. The action of the hands and arms is like a fountain which shoots up in a single jet, separates at the top, and falls to the earth in all directions. This exercise can also be done with the arms moving the opposite way, that is, swinging wide in a circle as you straighten up and coming together as you bend your knees again.

6.28 Ski and stretch Stand with the feet together. Drop down into a deep knee-bend, inclining the body forward and extending both arms to the rear, as in Slalom skiing. Straighten the legs and swing the arms forward and up above the head, leaning back as far as possible, and then drop into the knees-bend again.

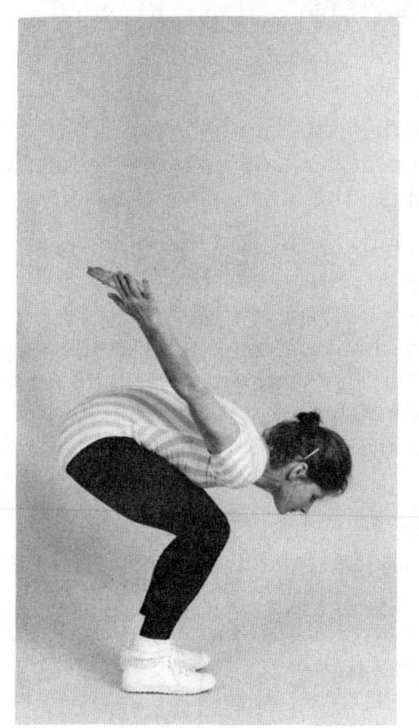

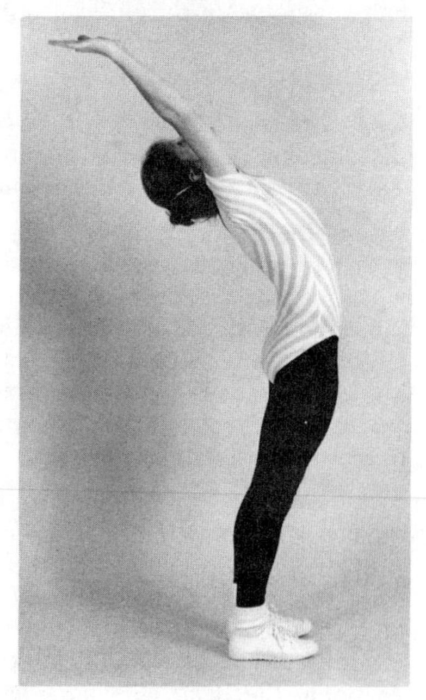

Exercise 6.28

6.29 Straight legs bend and stretch This is a similar exercise to the preceding one. Keep the legs straight, bend forward from the waist as far as possible, swinging both arms back and up. Straighten up, swinging the arms forward, and then above the head, bending as far back as possible.

6.30 Windmills There are a considerable number of arm-circling exercises which can be done in a standing position. All the swimming strokes can be imitated – front crawl, back-stroke, butterfly, and breast stroke. In addition, you can simply circle the arms at the side of the body in either direction, or in front of the body, moving both arms together or alternately. Most of the exercises can be done leaning forward from the waist.

6.31 Shoulder isolations Move each shoulder round in large exaggerated circles both forward and back either together or alternately. Also shrug both shoulders, bringing them close to the ears, then drop them again.

6.32 Shoulderblade touch Stand with both arms stretched wide, halfway between the direct front and side position. Keeping the arms held straight, move the shoulders back so as to touch the shoulderblades together.

6.33 Rib cage isolations Place both hands round the lower part of the rib cage. Move the rib cage from side to side and front to back. Take care to move the rib cage and not the hips.

6.34 Hip isolations Place both hands on the hips and lift each hip in turn up and out to the side. Push the buttock on the same side out with an exaggerated action. This can also be done lifting the arm on the opposite side of the raised hip, and pushing it high in the air, either with fingers extended or palm uppermost as if pushing up a low ceiling (see Fig. 6.4). Also try extending the arm on the same side as the raised hip. Variations include pushing the arm forward or to the side as the hip is moved.

6.35 Neck exercises Look round to the left as far as possible, then look round to the right, keeping the chin on the same plane. If necessary, use the fingers on the side of the chin to push it a little further. Do not jerk or flick the head around. Alternatively, look up high into the sky, keeping the jaws touching, then down to the ground, so that the chin touches the body. Other neck exercises are dropping the head to each side, ear towards the shoulder, and looking round to the side and up with the chin following a curving path (not an angular one). Go slowly on these exercises, otherwise you will feel dizzy.

6.36 Knee-bends There are a number of ways of working the legs in this movement. If your legs are supple enough, go into the full knee-bend, keeping thc heels on the floor. Otherwise, rise on to your toes as you go down. A strenuous form of the knee-bend is to come up from the deep squat into a jump in the air, then straight down again into the squat with no break in the movement. The arms can be held straight forward or out to the side, or with hands on the hips. Those who find the exercise hard can assist the upward movement by pushing down on their knees as they come up. Strong legs and good balance are required for the one-legged knee-bend (*strenuous*). Extend one leg forward, and go down into a deep knee-bend on the other leg, and then up again. You can hold on to something if you find it difficult to keep your balance. Once in the knee-bend position, there are a number of strenuous movements that can be performed. Fold the arms across the chest and kick each leg out to the front in turn, as in Russian dancing, or 'bunny hop' about, keeping the buttocks near the floor.

Feet astride

6.37 Sky reach Stand with the feet astride, both arms stretched above the head about shoulder-width apart. With both arms in the air, reach up higher with each arm in turn, stretching all that side of the body.

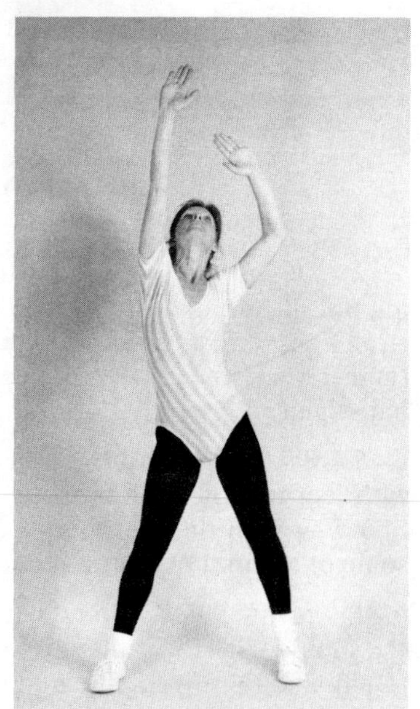

Exercise 6.37

6.38 Elbows to knees Start as for the previous exercise, arms high above the head. Turn the feet to point out diagonally. Go into a deep squat, and bring the arms down so that the elbows touch the knees. A variation of this exercise is to drop down into a half-squat position with the elbows about 12 inches (30 cm) away from the knees, and then rock the body from side to side so that the elbow touches the knee on the same side, with the foot on the opposite side rising on to the toes (*strenuous*).

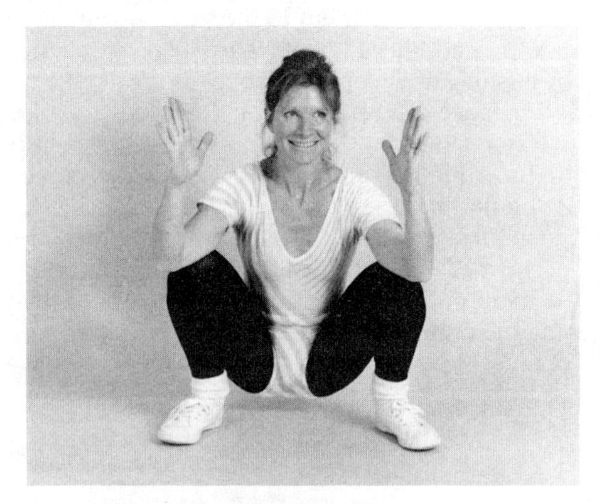

Exercise 6.38

6.39 Thigh stretch Stand with the feet wide apart and toes pointing out diagonally. Go into a half-squat or deeper, keep the back straight, and rest the hands on the hips. To stretch the inside of the thighs, rock the whole body from side to side, staying in the half-squat.

6.40 Windmills All the arm-circling exercises that can be done with feet together can be done with the feet astride (see page 93). Standing with the feet astride also gives a little more stability for some of the more vigorous ones.

6.41 Elbow touch Stand with the fingers of each hand touching the shoulder on the same side. Swing both elbows in to the centre to touch, and then swing them out. Variations are to rotate the points of the elbows in the air at the sides in either direction, or to include a push to the side, so the sequence is as follows: push to the side, touch the shoulders with the fingers, bring the elbows together and out, then push to the side, and so on.

6.42 Chest and arm tensing Extend both arms to the front, then fold in the forearms and grip the elbow with each hand. This is the starting position with the arms lifted up and folded. The exercise is to tense rhythmically all the muscles around the square formed by the folded arms and chest. This is a good bust exercise for women. A variation is to open the square slightly, with the hands holding lower down the forearms, and then swing the folded arms above the head and down again.

6.43 Side bends Extend both arms above the head, about shoulder-width apart. Holding them in that position, sway directly first to one side and then to the other. Breathe normally when you do this. Take care that you sway directly to the side, and do not bend forward from the hips. Imagine that you are standing between two sheets of glass and that no forward movement is possible. Less strenuous versions include: both hands held behind the head with fingers linked; one hand behind the head with the other hand on the hip (do not forget to reverse the hands to work the sides equally); both hands on the hips; and finally (the least strenuous) with both arms hanging down by the sides.

6.44 Forward bends This exercise works the lower back as well as the hamstrings. Keeping the legs straight, bend down to touch the floor between the legs, then straighten up and swing the arms above the head, bending back at the same time. An extra count can be put in when touching the floor either by touching further back between the legs or by touching the toes.

A variation is to bend down to touch the floor, then lift the trunk to a half-way position (parallel with the floor) flinging the arms out horizontally to the side. When the arms are flung out, try to flatten the back. Also repeat, touching either foot, coming up to that side and flattening the back. Caution: those with a history of back pain should not attempt to touch the floor, instead they should not go beyond the knee.

6.45 Trunk twists There are a number of exercises in this position which involve a twisting action of the trunk. A simple one is to bend forward from the waist, touching the left foot with the right hand, with the other arm swinging high in the air, and the eyes following it. Then repeat with the other arm, so this is done with a vigorous swing from side to side.

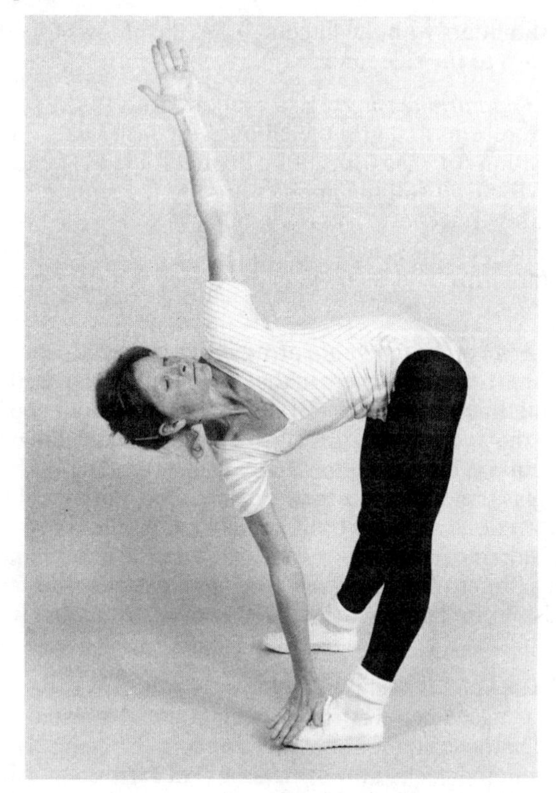

Exercise 6.45

Another way is to stand straight with the arms stretched out sideways, or arms folded, hands at the chest, and to swing the arms round to the side, twisting the upper body, and keeping the feet still. Variations on this are: to swing round to the left and punch the right fist out (or extend the fingers), and to swing to the left with the left hand resting on the left hip, and vice versa.

A complete trunk-twisting action is achieved by bending down to touch the floor with both hands, then swinging them up and round to the left, then bending right back with the hips pushed forward, taking the hands over the head, continuing round the circle to the right and down to the floor again, then back up the other way. Do this with legs straight or bent.

Crouching

Caution: all these exercises are strenuous and should not be attempted by the unfit or those with a history of back pain.

6.46 Squat thrusts Crouch down with hands on the floor about shoulder-width apart. This is a strenuous exercise which can be lightened either by raising the hands on finger-tips or by placing them on a low bench. Keeping the weight on the hands, thrust both legs back as far as they will comfortably go, then jump them forward again to bring the feet as near to the hands as possible. A slightly easier method is to jump one leg back at a time, bringing the other leg vigorously forward. A strenuous compound exercise known as the Burpee is to start in a standing position, then drop down into a crouch, make a squat thrust with both legs, then stand up again, and so on.

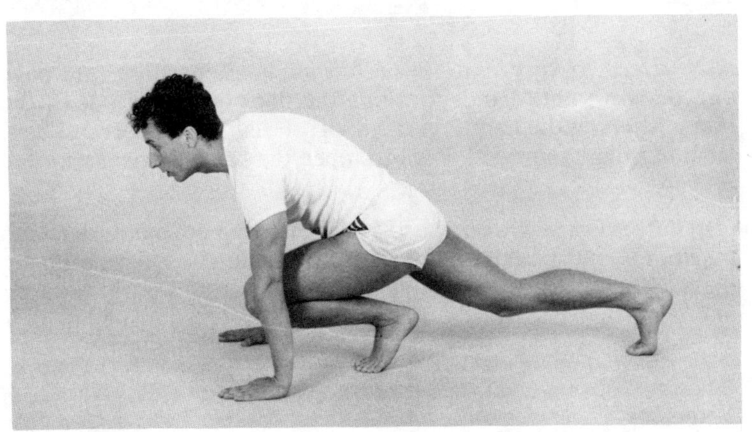

Exercise 6.46

6.47 Side jumps Crouching on the floor, hands touching the ground, jump with the legs together as far as possible to each side in turn.

6.48 Squat twists Crouch down in a deep squat. Spread the legs wide and point the toes out diagonally to the front. Staying in the deep squat, touch the left elbow to the right knee, and vice versa. If this is too easy, try touching the elbow to the opposite calf, or even down to the ankle.

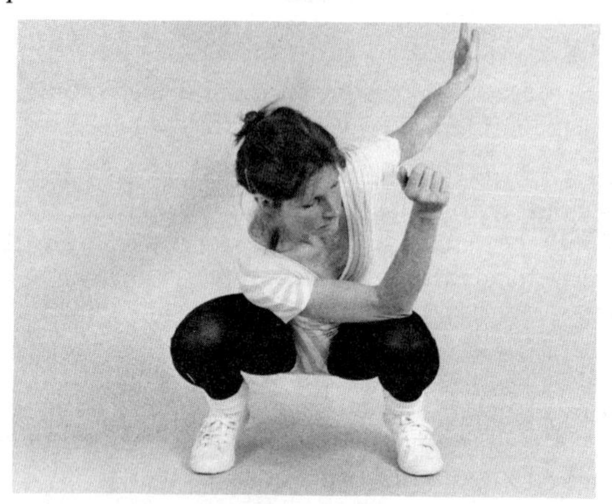

Exercise 6.48

6.49 Head to knee Go into a fencing-lunge position (see page 92), but with both hands touching the floor on either side of the body. Keeping the hands on the floor, straighten the forward bent leg and bring your head down to touch the knee. Repeat with the other leg.

6.50 Leg swings From the low crouch, with both hands touching the floor about shoulder-width apart, straighten both legs, bringing the backside as high as possible, and then from this position swing one leg up high backwards, pointing the toes. Repeat with the other leg.

Kneeling

6.51 Side swing Kneel up so that your thighs are vertical. Stretch both arms out to the front at shoulder height. Keeping the arms held out to the front, swing the buttocks over to one side, and sit on the floor. Kneel up again, and swing the buttocks over to the other side and sit on the floor.

6.52 Kowtow Start in the same kneeling position, then bend forward, bringing the head down to touch the floor. At the same time swing the arms back and up behind the body. As you bring the head down, the buttocks will come down on to the heels. Having touched the floor with the head, kneel up as high as possible, swinging the arms forward and up over the head, and lean back.

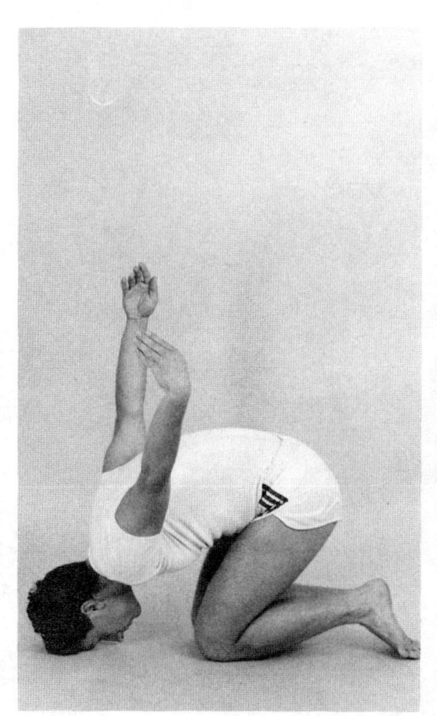

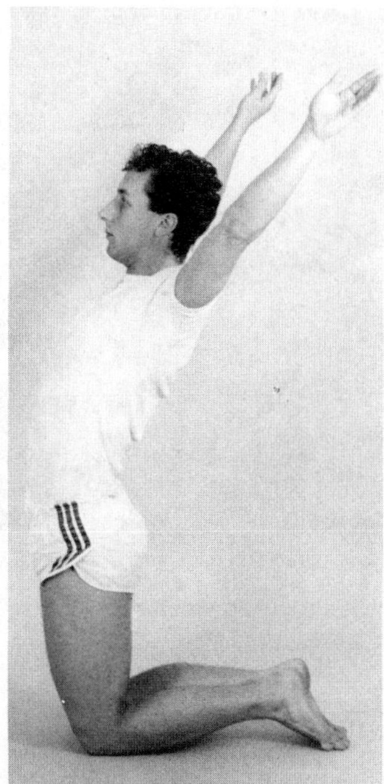

Exercise 6.52

6.53 Hip thrust There is not a lot of movement in this exercise; however it is a good one for the pelvic region. Kneel down on the heels, Japanese style, then lean back, taking the weight of the upper body on both arms placed about a foot to the rear. In that position push the hips forward and up as high as they will go, then drop them again, and repeat the whole movement.

Sitting

The sitting exercises are grouped in the following positions: sitting with legs together, sitting with legs spread wide, cross-legged sitting, and Indian-cross sitting.

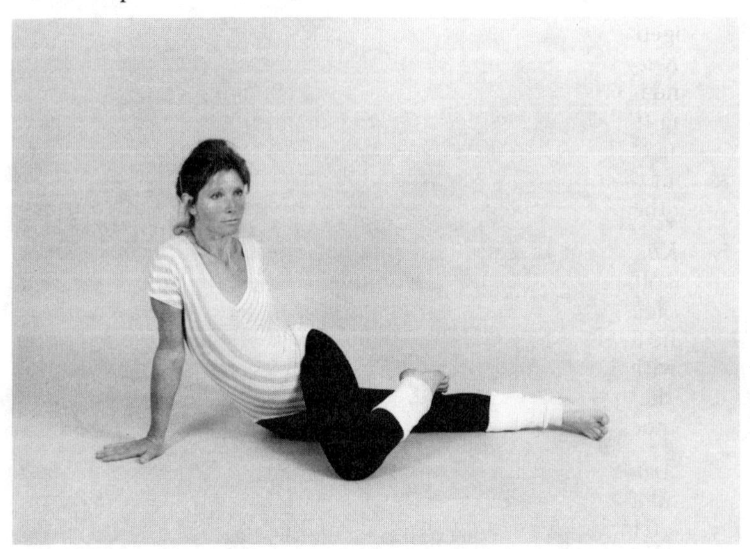

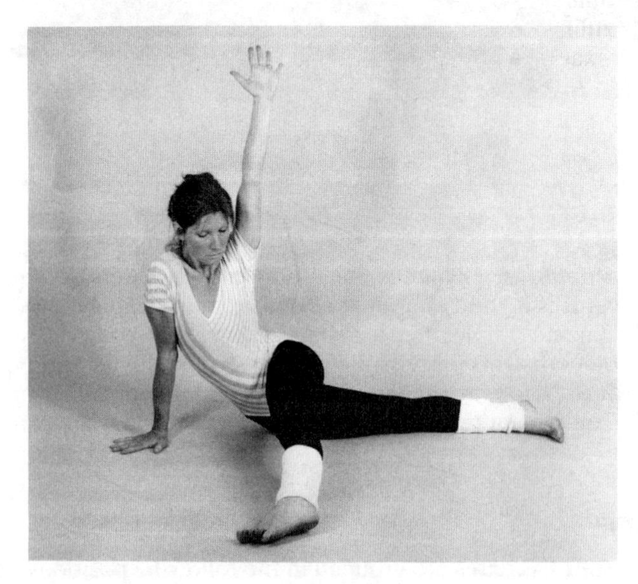

Exercise 6.55

Legs together

6.54 Knee rock Sit down with the feet extended straight out in front and both legs touching. Cross one leg over on top of the other. Keeping the legs in this position, rock from one side to the other, touching each knee to the ground in turn. In one direction it will be easy, but the other way requires a good stretch. After a few rocks, reverse the positions of the legs.

6.55 Knee and toe touch Sit with legs together stretched out in front. Rolling over on to the left buttock, bring the right knee over the left leg to touch the ground, then straighten the right leg and touch the toe to the ground as far round to the left as possible. Then repeat with the other leg. An extra movement with this exercise is to extend the arm on the same side of the body straight above the head, as the knee and toe touch.

6.56 Arm swing Start with legs together straight ahead. Slide one hand along the floor directly to the side as far as you can reach, and stretch the other arm in a curve over the head in the same direction the body is leaning. Repeat the other way.

6.57 Buttocks travel In the straight-legged sitting position, travel in a shuffling movement along the floor, forward and back, taking care to exaggerate the lifting action of the buttocks each time.

6.58 Rollover From the sitting position, twist round to the rear, and place both hands on the ground behind you. Continue the movement by rolling over on to the stomach and bending the legs. Keeping the trunk more or less in this position, let the momentum of the roll-over continue, and touch the feet to the ground. This gives quite a good twist to the hips. Roll back up to a sitting position and then roll over the other way. Note that the legs stay together throughout the exercise and bend into a right-angle half the way through.

Legs wide

6.59 Toe touch and swing Sit, spreading the legs wide with the backs of the knees pressed flat to the floor. Touch the toes of one foot with both hands, then swing both arms back the other way and up high to the opposite side, turning the head and upper body. Repeat a number of times to the same toe before switching to the other one. This exercise gives a considerable stretch to the sides of the trunk, and those with back trouble should only touch the knees.

6.60 Toe cross-swing Swing the right hand round to touch the left foot, then immediately swing the left hand round to touch the right foot, and so on. The other arm in each case is swung back behind you. Again, those with back trouble should only touch the knees.

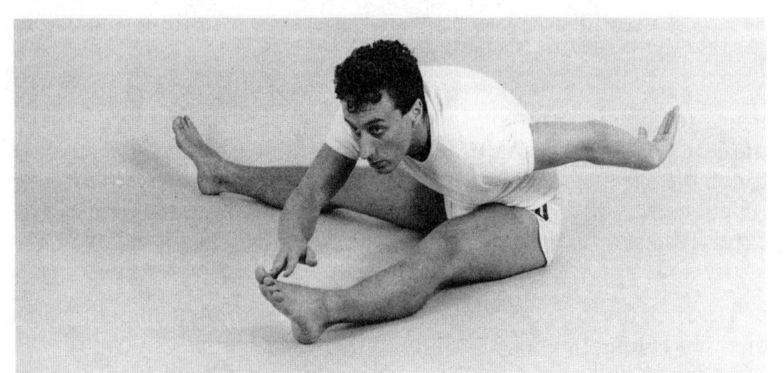

6.61 Seated twist Swing both arms right over to one side, placing both on the ground outside the legs, and bend the body to follow, so you touch the forehead to the ground.

6.62 Side-bend Hold the hands behind the head with fingers linked. Sway from side to side touching the elbow to the floor behind the knee or to the knee itself (strenuous). Also try touching the right elbow to the left knee, and vice versa.

A similar side-bending exercise can be done with one arm extended above the head, and swaying the body over to the opposite side, with the other arm extending across the abdomen in the other direction.

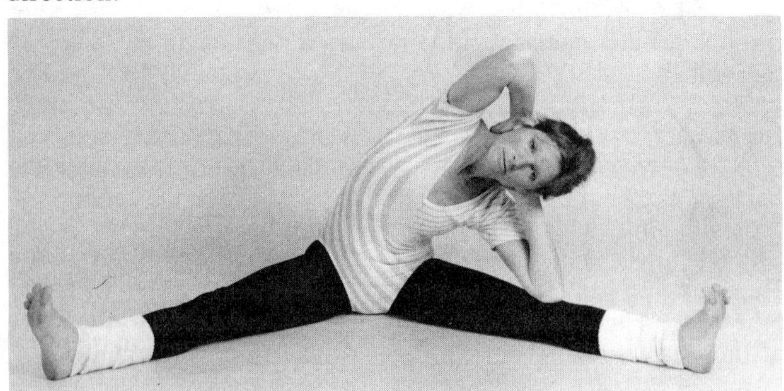

Cross-legged

6.63 Elbow to knee Sit cross-legged holding the hands behind the head with fingers linked. Twist round to the left and touch the right elbow to the left knee, straighten up, pushing the chest forward, then swing the other way. Take care not to just swing from side to side in a hunched position but to straighten up in between each elbow touch. This makes it a good posture exercise.

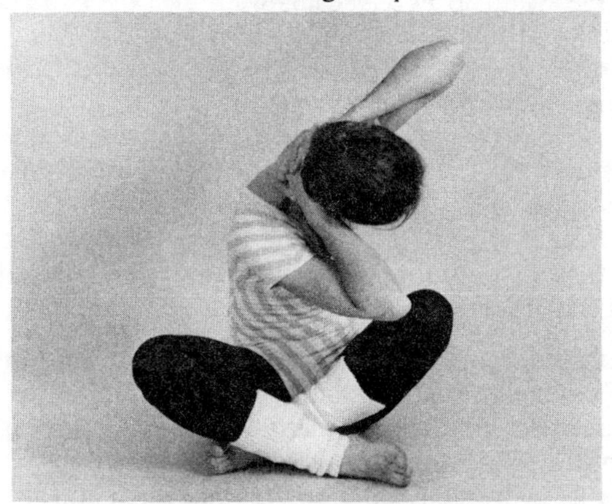

6.64 Crawl This exercise is a bit like the front crawl in swimming. Sitting in the cross-legged position, extend one arm to the front and the other to the rear, looking back over the rear shoulder, then swing the arms back the other way, lightly tapping the chest with both hands half-way.

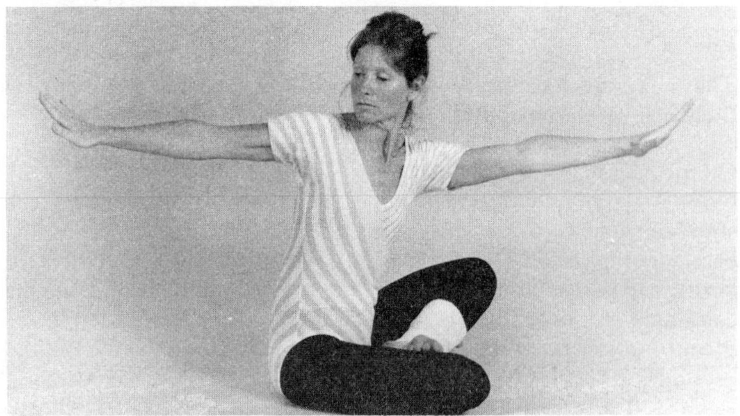

6.65 Side leg raise Lean over to the right and rest the right forearm on the ground. The other hand lightly touches the ground beside it. As you lean over, swing the left leg up straight and high in the air. Drop the leg back into the cross-legged position, and repeat on the other side. Point the toes.

6.66 Arm sway Sway over to the right, sliding the right arm along the floor and stretch a straight left arm over the head in the same direction. Repeat in the other direction.

Indian-cross

6.67 Swirl Cross one leg to the front as in the normal cross-legged position, but then cross the other leg behind to the rear. Tuck the feet close in to the body. Lean forward, extending both arms, then sway round in a circle, hands touching the floor for as long as possible. Also sway round in the other direction, and repeat, with the legs in the other position.

6.68 Reach and sway back Sit with the right leg folded to the front and extend the left leg straight to the rear. The right foot should almost be touching the left thigh. Drop the upper body forward and extend both arms along the floor to the front. Swing back up, resting the right hand on the right thigh and swing the left arm high up behind, turning the head and upper body to look at the hand. Repeat the movement a few times in this position, and then switch the legs round the other way.

Lying

These exercises are presented in the following sequence: lying on the back, on the side, and on the front.

On the back

6.69 Sit-ups This is a traditional exercise for working the stomach muscles, and is strenuous. There are several variations, the easiest being the half sit-up. Lie on the floor with the arms extended beside the body. Sit up, i.e., raise the upper body, until the fingers can touch the knee, then lie back on the floor, and repeat. If this is too strenuous, then bend the knees a little (keeping the feet on the ground).

The full sit-up can be done with the hands linked behind the head, folded on the chest, or stretched in front of the body. In most cases it will be necessary to anchor the feet under a piece of furniture so as not to over-balance. Lie flat on the back, with the head touching the floor, then sit up with the knees bent, and bend all the way forward.

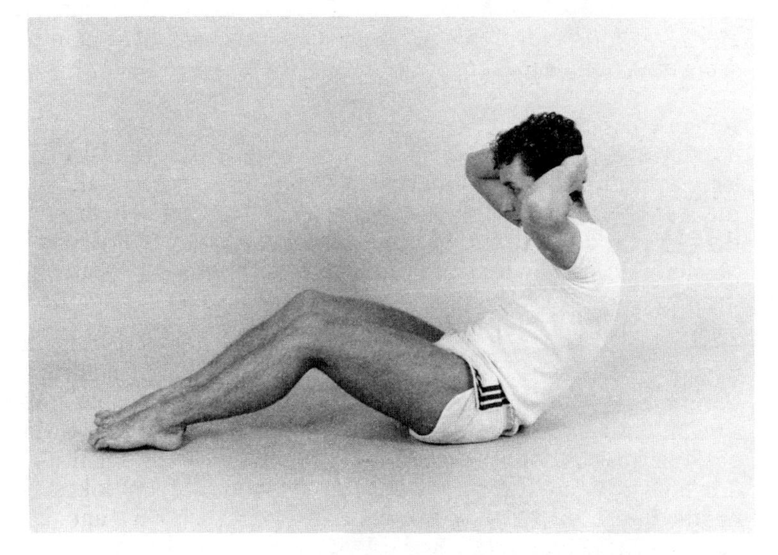

Exercise 6.69

Variations on the basic sit-up include: sitting up then twisting to the side; and making it more severe by raising the feet on an incline, and sitting up-hill, as it were. The very strong can do sit-ups virtually upside-down.

6.70 Crunches This is an exercise which eliminates the folding action at the hips and concentrates on the short, contracting action of stomach muscles. Lie close to a wall with the buttocks in the angle of the wall and the floor, and the legs up straight resting on the wall. Lie back, touching the head to the floor, then reach up with the hands to touch the feet and also try to touch the head to the knees. A slightly more strenuous version of this is to do it without the wall holding the legs up vertical and straight. A chair can also be used, in which case the lower leg rests on the chair. The arm position can also be varied as with the ordinary sit-up.

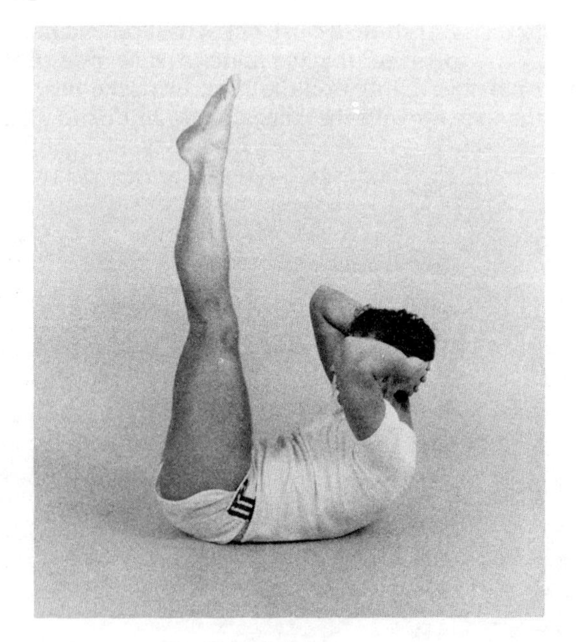

Exercise 6.70

6.71 Sit-backs This is an exercise which works the muscles of the stomach in an unusual way. One of the functions of the stomach muscles is to work like a corset, that is, to hold the area together. This exercise mimics that function. Hook your feet under a piece of furniture, fold your arms across your chest and lean back at about 45 degrees. Simply hold this position for as long as possible. If you start to tremble, stop. Harder versions of this are: to hold the position further back, and to change the arm position, either linking the hands behind the head or stretching the arms above the head in a line with the body and looking at the ceiling. Dig your fingers into the stomach while doing the exercise and you will see how firm the muscles have to be.

6.72 Leg raises The stomach can also be worked from the opposite direction, that is, by raising the legs instead of the upper body (strenuous). Lie on the floor, and keeping the legs together and straight, raise them off the ground and swing them up over towards the head. When swinging them back to the floor, try to stop just short of the floor before repeating the exercise. If necessary, anchor the body by holding wall-bars or a low piece of furniture at arms length. Those who find it difficult to lift straight legs can try bending the legs and bringing the knees up towards the head and lifting the hips off the ground. This is not an exercise for those with lower back trouble, however.

As with the ordinary sit-up, this exercise can be made more strenuous by doing it on an incline (feet lower than the head) or hanging vertically from a beam.

6.73 Jack-knife This is a strenuous stomach exercise which is a combination of sit-up and leg lift. Lie stretched out on the floor, with your arms extended along the floor above the head. Sit up *and* raise the legs in one movement, and touch the toes. Try to keep the legs straight. Lie back and lower the legs in one movement, and repeat the exercise. It will take a short while to get the hang of the balance in this exercise.

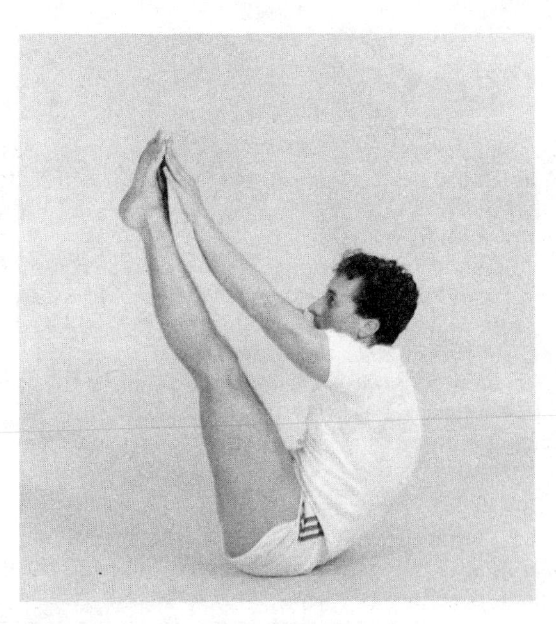

Exercise 6.73

6.74 Leg swings Lie on the ground and bring both knees up towards the chest. Stretch both arms out to the side along the ground. Keeping the knees together and legs bent, swing them over from side to side touching the ground each time. This will give the trunk a good stretch. Try to keep the shoulders in contact with the ground throughout the exercise.

A more strenuous version of this exercise is to start with the legs held together, vertical and *straight*, and to swing them from side to side, lightly touching the ground on each side.

6.75 Scissors Prop yourself up on your elbows from the lying position and lift both legs in the air keeping them straight. In this position move them vertically up and down in fairly small scissor-like movements. Also raise and lower the legs as you make the scissoring movements. A similar exercise is to cross the legs over and under, while lowering them gradually to the floor. Avoid this exercise if you have any lower back pain problems.

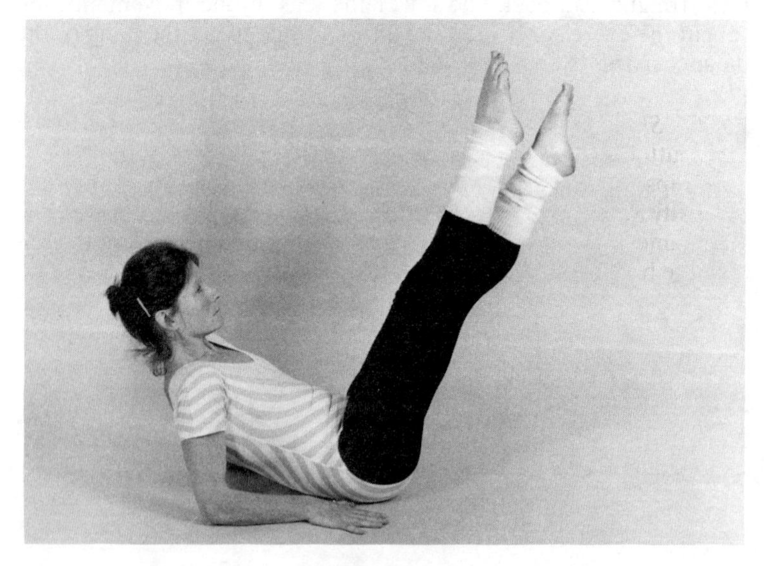

Exercise 6.75

6.76 Heel kicks Lie on the ground with the head off the floor, hands touching behind the head, fingers linked. In this position, move the legs in a reverse bicycling action, that is to say, pedal in the opposite direction to that of a bike, but pull the toes back and kick just over the ground with the heels. Imagine you are kicking something with your heels that is three or four inches off the ground.

A similar, but harder, exercise is to touch each knee with the opposite elbow as the knee comes up each time. This will give a little extra twist to the trunk each time.

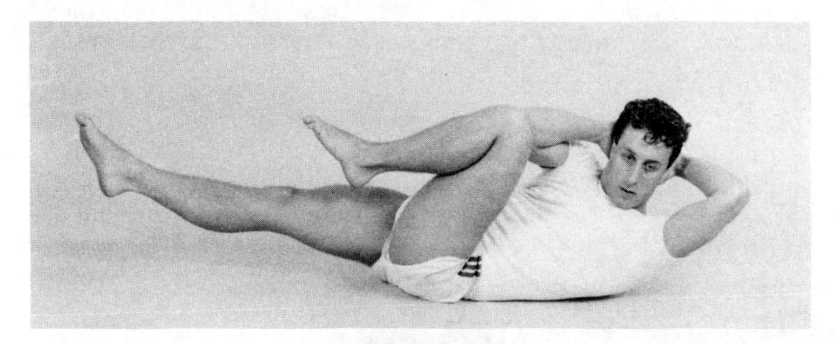

Exercise 6.76

6.77 Shoulder bridge Lying on the back, walk the feet close into the buttocks until the hips rise off the floor. From this position, lift the hips up as high as they will go, and lower them to the floor. Usually this is done with the knees apart, however as a variation, try the same lift with the knees together. This is an excellent exercise for the buttocks.

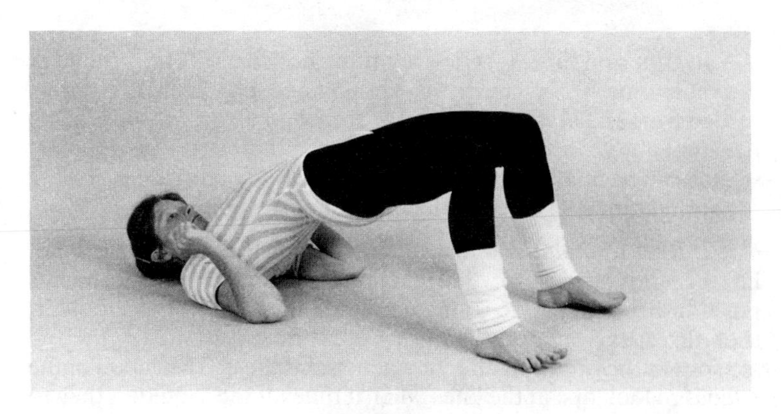

Exercise 6.77

On the side

6.78 Side leg raises Lie on your side on the ground, one leg on top of the other, your head supported by your hand. Raise and lower the top leg, either pointing the toes or pulling the foot and toes hard back. When lowering the leg, touch the other one lightly – do not crash it down or rest it.

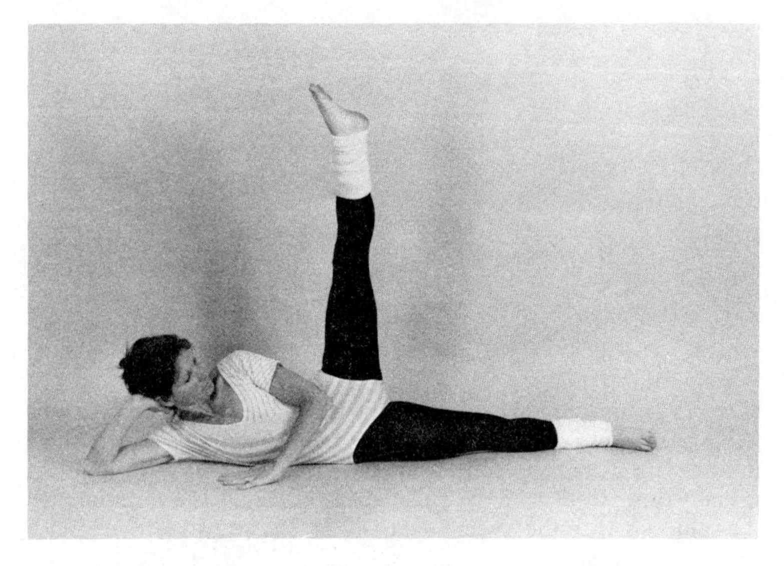

Exercise 6.78

Variations on this exercise are: lifting both legs off the ground at the same time (this is strenuous, with limited movement), lowering the leg from the high position to the front and up again, and circling the upper leg, with the foot circling in either direction. A good stretch can be made by catching hold of the foot or ankle and pulling the straightened leg over the head as far as possible.

6.79 Knee to shoulder Instead of propping the head on the hand, lift the body slightly so that it is propped on the elbow. In this position bring the knee of the upper leg in to touch the shoulder, then thrust the leg away, pointing the toes and stretching the top arm out in the opposite direction across the chest. The action of the head is to look first at the knee when it touches the shoulder, then to look at the hand when it stretches out to the side.

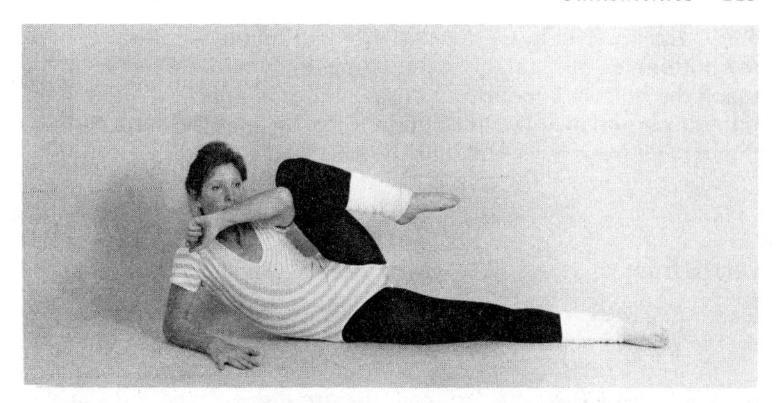

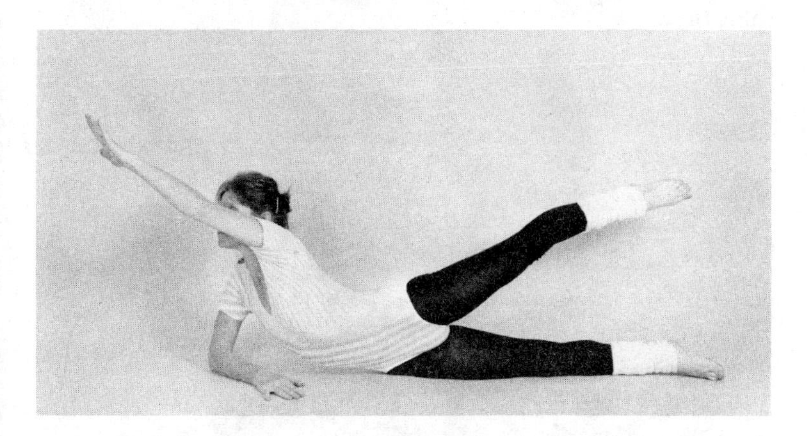

Exercise 6.79

6.80 Elbow to floor and lift In this exercise, lift the body even higher than in the previous one, and support it on a straight arm. Bend the top leg, and place the foot on the floor in front of the knee of the bottom leg, which is straight. From this position, first place the elbow of the free arm on the floor (this is a good hip stretch), next lift the hips off the floor as high as they will go, balancing on two feet and one hand, and at the same time swing the other arm over the head and stretch it to the side. Lower to the ground, then lift the *bottom* leg to touch the rear of the knee about it, with the knee. Repeat a few times, then change to the other side.

6.81 Leg flick Lie on the side propped up on one elbow. Bend the bottom leg into a right angle. Bring the foot of the top leg up to touch the bottom knee. From this position flick the foot straight up into the air and over the head making the leg as straight as possible, then take it back down to touch the knee again.

On the front

6.82 Leg raises Lie on the stomach, with the palms of the hands on the ground beneath the shoulders. Lift one leg as high as it will go, lower, then lift the other leg (strenuous). This exercise can also be done lifting the body up from the ground with the arms at the same time.

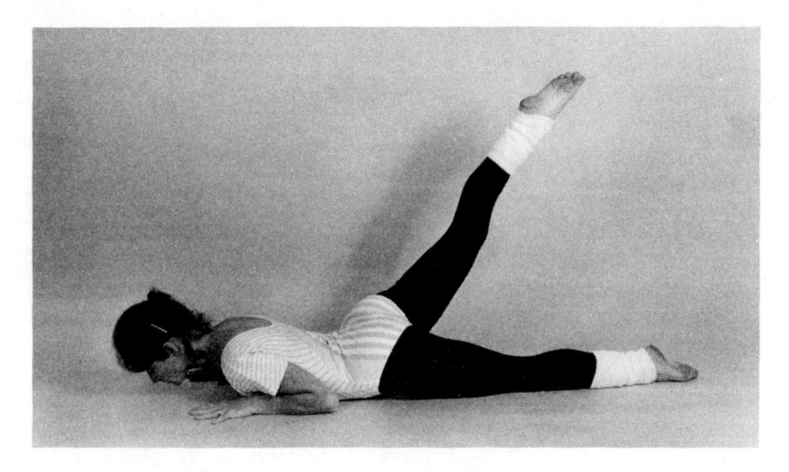

Exercise 6.82

6.83 Back arches Link the hands across the small of the back. Push the hands down towards the buttocks, and at the same time lift both legs and the upper body off the ground in a curve. Hold for a second or two, then rest and repeat. Try to lift the thighs and chest completely off the ground (strenuous). This exercise can also be done with the arms in different positions. Try holding the hands behind the head, stretched out to the side or forwards in a line with the body.

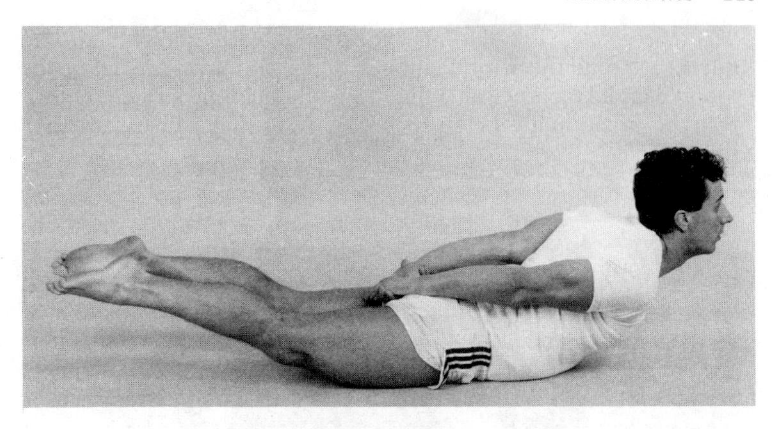

Exercise 6.83

6.84 Upper body raise This is not a strenuous exercise, but it will help to loosen the lower back. Place the hands palm down beneath the shoulders. Raise the upper body as high as it will go, just using the back muscles, then gently push higher using the arms, and look up at the ceiling. Try to keep the hips in contact with the floor during the exercise. Stretch can be increased by gradually moving the hands nearer to the hips.

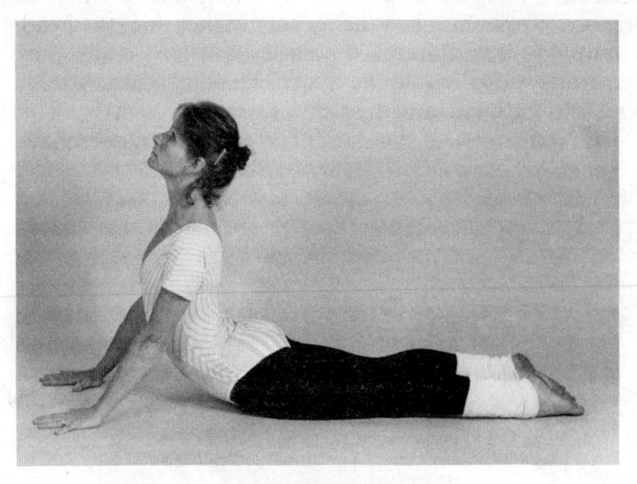

Exercise 6.84

6.85 Hip raise Lie flat on the ground with the toes tucked underneath, and the arms bent back, so the forearms are flat on the ground with hands alongside the shoulders pointing straight ahead. From this position lift the buttocks as high as they will go, and then lower.

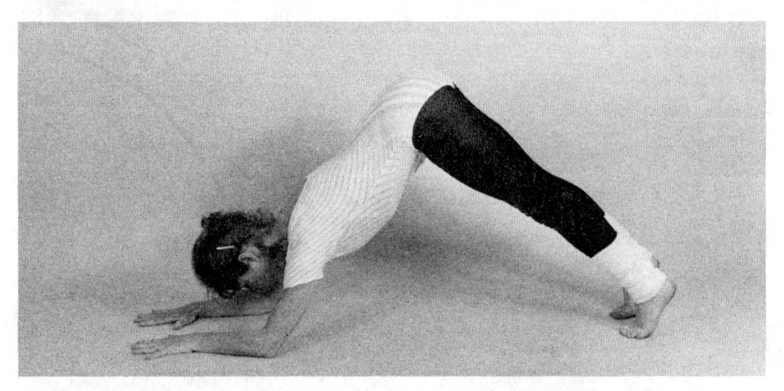

6.86 Press-ups (push-ups) This is a strenuous arm exercise that can be done in a variety of ways. Those who have very little arm strength can practise the move standing, against a wall. As they get stronger, the angle of the body can be changed, so that it is done against a low piece of furniture such as a table. The exercise becomes more strenuous as the body is held horizontally, and then even more strenuous when the feet are higher than the head.

When lying horizontally, the easiest way to do the press-up is while resting the knees on the floor. The body is kept straight from the knees to the head, and the arms press the body up from the floor, and lower it again. The standard press-up is to support the body on

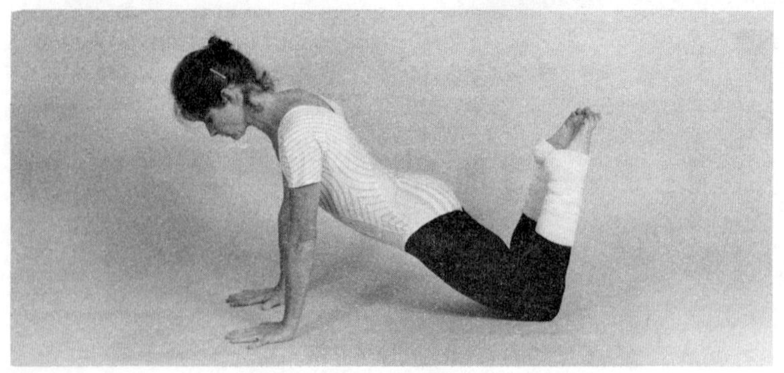

the balls of the feet and the hands. The entire body is held straight, and the arms press the body up from the floor to full arms' length. When lowering the body to the floor, touch the nose or chest to the ground, and do not sag in the middle. This way the arms are exercised through the full range of movement.

The hands can be positioned anywhere from under the chest to wide out to the side. Usually the hands are shoulder-width apart. The exercise can be made more strenuous by pushing up vigorously from the floor so that the hands leave the floor momentarily at full reach, and then interposing a clap, or touching the opposite shoulder.

6.87 Cat-dip Start in the standard press-up position, but with the feet about two feet apart, then sway back so that the buttocks rise much higher than the shoulders. At this point the arms and trunk should be in a straight line. From here dip the upper body down so that the nose drops down to the ground roughly in a line with the hands, then skims forward and up as the buttocks and hips drop close to the ground. At this point the movement is very like a cat stretching. As the buttocks drop, the arms straighten, and then the buttocks are lifted high again to the starting position, and the movement is repeated. The whole movement is a continuous dip, press and lift, making sure that the knees do not rest on the floor at any point, and is a strenuous exercise.

6.88 Thigh raise Lie flat on the floor, bend and lift the lower legs up, toes pointing to the ceiling. From this position, lift the thighs off the ground, and push the toes up to the ceiling. The legs stay bent throughout the movement. There is a limited range of movement in this exercise, but it is good for the buttocks.

6.89 Butterflies Lie flat on the stomach, but put the hands under the hips so as to get the middle body just clear of the ground. Stretch the legs back, pointing the toes, then, lifting them off the ground a few inches, cross them over and under, keeping the legs straight.

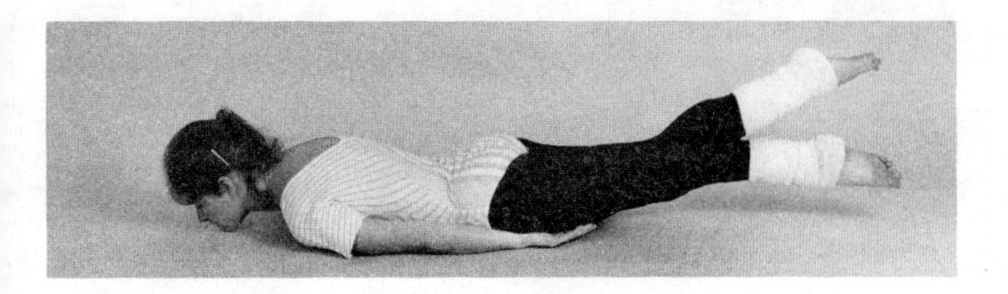

All-fours

6.90 Leg swings In the all-fours position, knees on the ground, body supported on straight arms, swing one knee in under the body and try to touch the head with the knee. Swing the leg back and high up into the air, pointing the toes and lifting the head high at the same time. This is a very good trunk exercise.

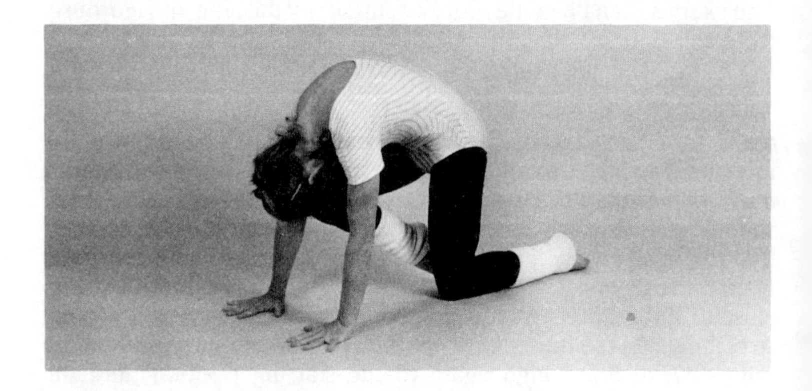

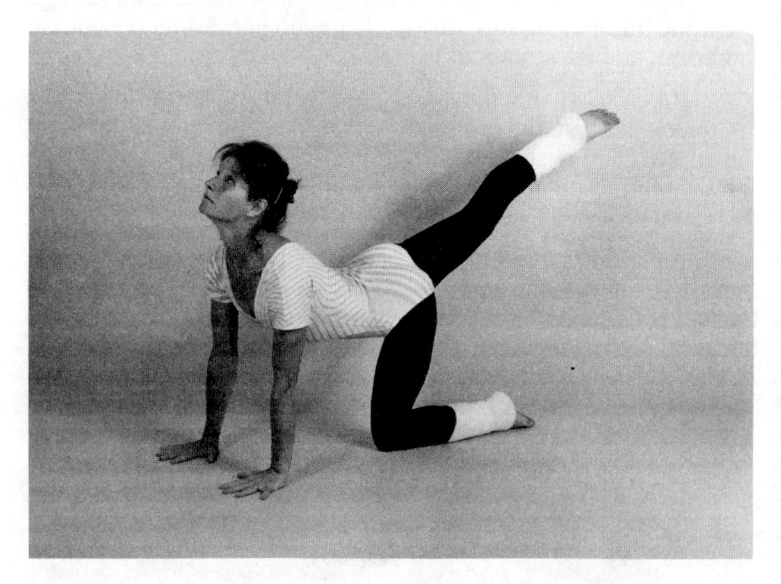

Exercise 6.90

6.91 Side leg raise From the all-fours position, lift one knee slightly off the ground, then lift the bent leg up to the side as high as it will go, and lower.

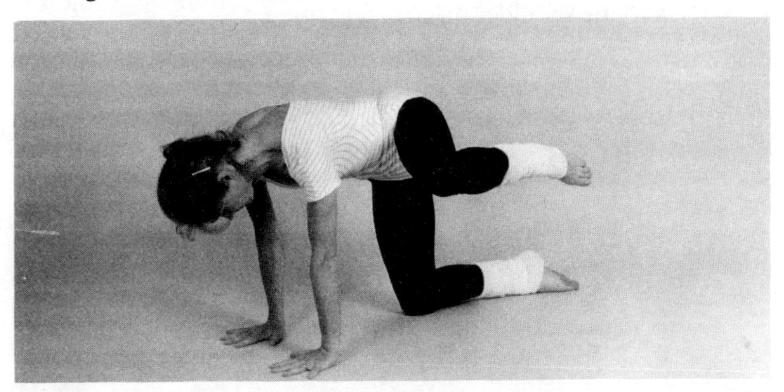

Exercise 6.91

6.92 High flicks Again from the all-four position, lift one knee as high up and out as possible. Holding the thigh high, flick the lower leg back and forwards vigorously, trying to kick the bottom each time.

6.93 Side, cross and lift Beginning on all fours, stretch one leg out straight to the side then swing it round behind to the other side, crossing over the other leg. From this crossed position swing the leg high in the air pointing the toes. Return to the starting position with knees together and repeat with the other leg. When crossing the leg take care to cross it as far over as possible. This is a good buttocks exercise.

6.94 Humping In the all-fours position, hump the back as high as it will go, dropping the head at the same time. Then lift the head and drop the back, trying to create a hollow in the middle. Take care to keep the arms straight throughout and try to achieve a rhythmical undulating movement of the back.

6.95 Side-swings Bring the knees tight together and lift the feet off the floor. Swing the feet from side to side, and as the feet come to each side, bend the trunk and look at them. This flexes the body in the opposite plane to the humping exercise. Try to achieve a rhythmical swing from side to side.

6.96 Mule kick Bring one knee forward so as to touch the shoulder. From this position, kick the leg strongly back parallel with the floor, either pointing the toes or pulling them back. Pull the knee back to the shoulder on each repetition.

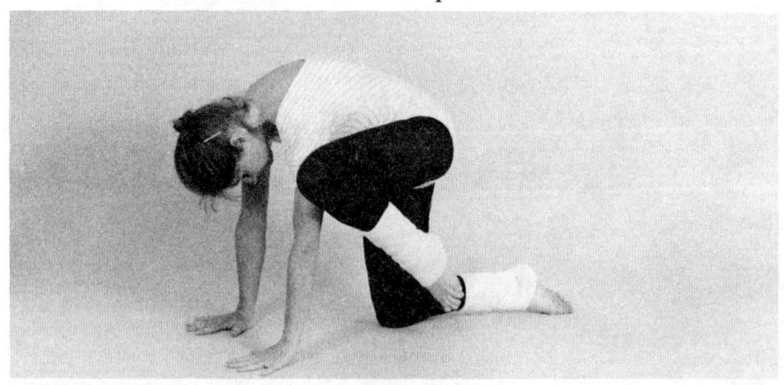

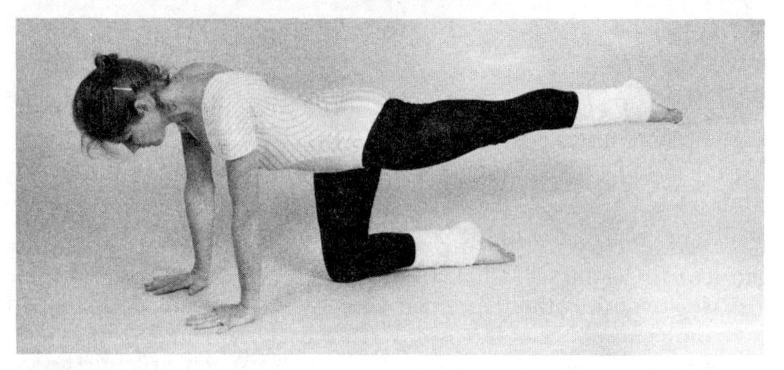

Most of these exercises are suitable for women. Several of them, such as press-ups, are more difficult. Men who want a more vigorous workout can select the tougher exercises and do much higher repetitions. Men should try all the exercises since many of them are deceptive, especially the dance-type movements. Supple hips and legs are required and the average stiff male will find them very strenuous.

In addition to the exercises in this chapter, there are many more of a similar nature using light equipment. For example, there are ballet exercises holding on to a barre, and many using sticks, hoops, ball, ropes and clubs. In addition to this there are exercises that can be done with a partner. The complete range of exercises, with or without equipment or partner, is endless.

7

Suppleness: Basic Yoga

Suppleness is an important but often overlooked aspect of general fitness, especially in men. If the body is stiff, it cannot assume a balanced posture in all activities, and imbalance leads to fatigue from unnecessary muscular effort and often to permanent tension and pain. Unless we deliberately stretch the body, it tends to stiffen as we grow older, from early childhood onwards. The muscles tend to contract inwards in stressful situations and this tight posture can become habitual if our mental attitude is negative; feelings of unhappiness, conflict, or inferiority result in postures in which bent or curved positions predominate.

The life-style of many people today is not conducive to an alert, open posture. Apart from mental stress, physical inactivity contributes to the stiffening process. Even if one is undergoing fitness training of some kind, this does not always bring with it an awareness of good posture, and the greater part of one's life may still involve sitting awkwardly in badly designed chairs or assuming a bad posture due to conditions of work (for example, using the arms and hands at a work surface which is not at the ideal height). In fact, there are many sports and physical activities which cause certain parts of the body to become stiffer, a common example being the tightening effect on the hamstrings of running and bicycling. Many activities involve the development of certain groups of muscles while neglecting others, and there are very few sports, if any, which strengthen or stretch the body evenly. Thus it is very important for the players to stretch the body deliberately and systematically, to counteract any imbalance caused by the sport itself.

Apart from the feeling of relaxation, energy and well-being that is generated by stretching, there are other benefits for the athlete. Keeping the muscles, ligaments and joints flexible helps to prevent injury and long-term damage, including arthritis. The increased range of movement gained from greater mobility also helps to improve skill in one's particular sport. This is easily seen in a sport such as judo which has a very large number of moves and techniques, requiring the body to adopt many different positions, but it is also important in sports with a more limited range of movement, such as running. Running tends to tighten both the hamstrings and the quadriceps, gradually restricting the freedom of the knee joint itself. A well-stretched muscle also probably has more power of contraction than a tight one which cannot stretch very far.

Yoga stretching

Probably the best and most systematic way of stretching is through the yoga postures. There are literally hundreds of postures in yoga, but regularly practising even a dozen of the most basic will bring into play every joint and muscle of the body. The systematic nature of yoga means that a person's individual weaknesses are immediately and clearly revealed, while practising the postures correctly will start to improve these weak points. Unlike other forms of exercise, where the aim is to develop a skill or to win competitively, in yoga the aim is the work on oneself, and there is no external goal. Thus, whereas in sport, or even dance, a weakness can be compensated for by overdeveloping another part of the body, in yoga this kind of 'cheating' does not occur, because it is the weak points which represent the way to progress. Thus in the yoga stretches, you are confronted with yourself as you really are and this must be accepted before you can improve. The effect of the postures is always to bring into balance the different parts of the body, and to lead to a harmony between body and mind. Both sides of the body, left and right, are worked evenly, with special attention paid to the stiffer or weaker side. The top half of the body is loosened and stretched with as much attention as the lower half (there are many other programmes for increasing suppleness which work extensively on the hips and legs while neglecting the shoulders and upper part of the spine). In fact, with continuing practice, the correspondences between the different parts of the body become more and more apparent. Paradoxically, the more freedom of movement that can be obtained in the individual parts of the body, and the more it becomes possible to isolate movements, the clearer the relationships become, and the unity of the whole is more obvious.

Especially important is the way in which yoga works on the spine. The spine is not only the backbone of our structure, but a part of the central nervous system from which all the main nerves of the body emanate. The health of our nerves depends largely on the health of the spine. With our upright posture, compared with the horizontal spines of animals, the pressure of gravity on the spine is very great. The structure of the spine has adapted to withstand this, but without deliberate stretching there is considerable compression on the inter-vertebral discs. The lower, or *lumbar* spine is particularly vulnerable to strain, since it is very flexible, and is not protected by the bony structure of the pelvis or the rib-cage.

When they are correctly done, all the yoga postures involve stretching and strengthening the different parts of the spine. It is the combination of *stretching* and *strengthening* which is significant. For example, many people may have apparently very strong muscles in the lumbar area, but these muscles may be shortened from compression and lack of stretching. This constitutes an overall weakness of the back, and such a person may well eventually suffer from back pain. In yoga, the holding of a pose with the muscles stretched, strengthens the muscles at their most extended position.

Apart from its systematic nature, it is the actual *process* of yoga stretching which sets it apart from other limbering and suppling exercises. Yoga stretching is slow and smooth, and achieved gradually over a period of time. Every pose, once attained, is held for a period lasting from twenty seconds to ten or fifteen minutes, depending on the pose and the experience of the person practising. Trying to stretch by jerking or bouncing only invokes what the physiologists call the 'stretch reflex', which results in a further contraction and tightening of the muscles that are being stretched. When a stretch is held for a half a minute or so, the initial stretch reflex disappears as the stretch is maintained and muscle activity is reduced, resulting in true muscular relaxation.

This process has many simultaneous effects. The mind is naturally involved because to hold a stretch without resistance requires considerable concentration. As the body is being stretched to its limit, and the mind concentrates hard, there is a letting go of unnecessary mental activity and tension as well as physical. As your limits are revealed, and your reactions to these limitations are observed, a process of self-discovery and acceptance begins. In the true practice of yoga, the mind must stay in the present and cease striving after a future goal. This has a mentally relaxing effect, and also a liberating and stimulating one, for when there is acceptance and relaxation, there is a letting-go of the blocks (mental and physical – they reflect each other) which are preventing you from going further.

So, in yoga, no movement is ever forced; it is a process not of imposing a condition on the body but of releasing the obstructions which prevent the body from moving freely. The whole attitude required and engendered by yoga practice can have a therapeutic effect on people who are tense from the pressures of day-to-day life, and also on those engaged in competitive sports, where anxiety or ambition can inhibit efficient performance.

Yoga is not only an invaluable complementary activity for other types of exercise, but is also an excellent starting point for those who have lost touch with their bodies through years of neglect and inactivity. Because nothing is forced, there is no danger of injury. Because yoga develops strength and suppleness evenly, a balance is cultivated. The weak person will gradually increase in strength and the stiff person in suppleness; the aggressive person will relax, and the timid person will gain confidence, and so on. Perhaps good health can be defined as a perfect balance or harmony of the body and personality, of the whole person. Yoga is a system which always leads towards a position of balance, of being centred, whatever the starting point.

Thus it is clear that yoga is more than an efficient system of developing suppleness. The very process which makes it so successful as a means of becoming supple also brings many psychological benefits. The connection between mind and body becomes more and more apparent, and with this comes the ability to 'tune in' to your body, and so to be able to listen to its needs and signals. One example of this is the way in which your eating habits can be affected. You are less likely to overeat at any one meal or to eat from habit rather than hunger; appetite becomes the true guide to food intake that it should be. Many overweight people have found that they lose weight gradually on starting yoga and that their weight then stabilises. Eating ceases to be an automatic response to stress or depression. Living truly in your body in this way brings a new kind of confidence and sense of self; you become gradually less dependent on external influences for your well-being, and develop a kind of 'inner strength'.

All these benefits come from *regular* practice, and regular stretching. It is not necessary to practise for a long time every day, but you should try to do something. Although a session lasting an hour and a half is obviously very beneficial, five or ten minutes a day is infinitely better than none at all. Moreover, once you are familiar with the basic yoga stretches, it is surprising how easily and to what an extent they can become incorporated into your everyday life. As the body gets used to stretching, the way you stand and walk, and your posture generally will improve. There will be times when you will instinctively stretch the spine, or the backs of the legs, or the shoulders or neck, because the body seems to need it. You will become more aware of the way you make movements such as bending over to pick things up, or using your arms in activities such as cleaning, or even writing. In the postures which are described in this chapter, suggestions are made as to how to incorporate some of them into your daily life.

How and when to practise

All these stretching exercises should be done on an empty stomach, so allow a few hours after a main meal. If you practise in the morning, which is a good time, take a light breakfast. If you are combining the stretching with another sport, do your stretching exercise after playing, when the body is warm, and finish with complete relaxation in the *Corpse Pose* (see page 149). Early evening before supper is another good time for a regular practice.

Clothes should be as light and unrestricting as possible. Tights, tracksuit trousers, or stretchy shorts are best for the legs; there should be nothing constricting around the waist or crutch. Feet should be bare. T-shirts or leotards should allow complete freedom of movement. Cotton is the best material – nylon is harsh and slippery – and bare skin is best of all if the weather is warm enough. The texture and movement of the skin are important in the yoga exercises, and when the skin is encased in a corset of nylon, it tends to lose its sensitivity. If possible, practise in a warm, airy place. For some postures a blanket is necessary, and for others it is useful to have some clear wall space and a bar or some kind of ledge at about waist height that you can use as a support (a chest of drawers or a table would do very well. For stiffer people, a firm length of webbing or cloth is an invaluable aid to stretching correctly, for example, it can be looped round the feet to help in bending forward.

Only a few of the basic postures, with a few variations, are dealt with here. They all contribute towards the stretching and strengthening of the legs and spine, and to increasing the flexibility of the hip, knee and shoulder joints, as well as working the feet and hands and improving balance and symmetry in general.

The standing postures are the most fundamental, because they develop mobility and strength in the legs and feet, and improve your awareness of your centre of gravity and balance, as well as making the hips more flexible and stretching the spine. Anyone, however weak or stiff, can attempt the basic standing postures and get some benefit from them. Obviously it is sensible to learn to stand up straight on your feet before attempting to balance on your head or do advanced forward-bending or back-bending work, as the relationship between legs, pelvis and spine can be experienced and adjusted in the standing poses. The inverted postures form another basic group. There are many benefits from being upside-down, reversing the effects of gravity, but it is important that the body should be properly aligned, hence the importance of practising the standing poses and learning to *feel* when the body is straight. The Dog Pose is a fundamental, self-contained posture, combining the effects of standing and inverted poses and giving a thorough stretch to the whole body. The floor poses are particularly for stretching and twisting the spine, and increasing flexibility in the hips, knees, ankles and shoulders; these positions should not be attempted without practice of the standing postures.

These postures are all designed to be held for a period ranging from a few seconds to a few minutes, depending on the individual pose and the expertise of the practitioner. When attempting them for the first time, hold them for not more than twenty seconds, and less if you find that you are under strain. While you are holding a pose, you should breathe normally; *never* hold your breath. Usually, movement into a pose is done on the exhalation, unless it involves bringing the head up from a lowered position, in which case it is better to inhale to avoid feeling dizzy. When in doubt, just breathe normally. Keeping the breath relaxed while holding a posture helps you to approach the poses in a relaxed frame of mind. Even the most strenuous postures should be done with an inner quietness, so that it is possible to concentrate and observe the body attentively. When doing the poses, you should be still, steady and firm, but never rigid. While holding a pose you should always be seeking to stretch and extend further, to create movement and space where there is stiffness and tightness.

Make sure that you work both sides of the body evenly, holding postures for the same length of time on the left and the right. Try to be aware of the back of the body as much as the front; because we look forwards, we tend to be much more aware of what is happening in front. Do not be ambitious in the way you work at the postures, but also do not lose hope if you find them difficult. Those that are the hardest for you should be practised with the most application. Even those that come more easily can always be improved. Precision is extremely important, so read the instructions right through before starting, and look at the illustrations carefully.

For many yoga practioners the core of their practice is the regular work they do at home. Yoga is a process of self-discovery and self-awareness and, although a good teacher is always necessary, it is essentially an individual journey. However, it is vital for the beginner to start correctly and at this stage a teacher is indispensable. Most local education authorities run evening or day classes under qualified teachers. After your introduction to the yoga world you will hear of other or more advanced teachers. The first teacher you encounter may not suit you and it is a good idea to try different teachers provided they teach the same style or type of yoga. The type of yoga described in this book is Hatha Yoga in the Iyengar style.

Four basic stretches

These basic stretches can be done any time, especially the first two, which can be done at the kitchen sink while waiting for the kettle to boil, or in any other similar situation. They are all excellent preparation for the other postures and should form the start of your practice.

7.1 For spine and legs

(*a*) Stand with feet parallel, hip-width apart, facing a wall or work top. Bend from the hips and place your hands on the wall. You should make a straight line from hands to buttock bones, parallel to the floor, so make sure that you are far enough from the wall to stretch the arms, shoulders and back properly. Keep your knees straight and lift the hips away from the floor and away from the wall so that both legs and back are well stretched. The spine should neither hump up nor hollow down, but remain quite flat, so feel with one hand to check the position of your back. Imagine that you are making more space between all the vertebrae. As you stretch, you may need to move your feet a little further from the wall to keep the legs perpendicular.

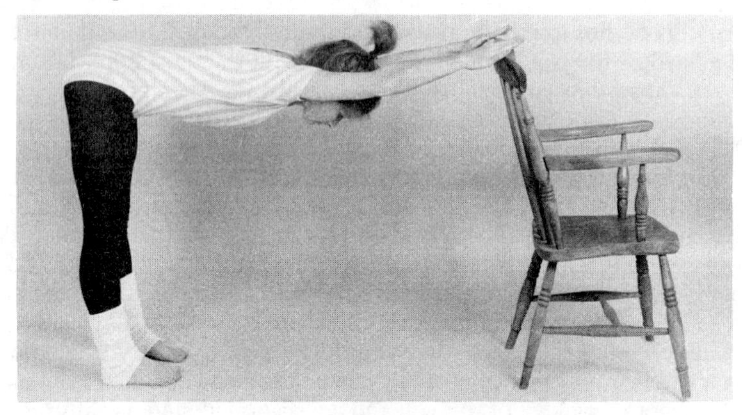

Exercise 7.1

(*b*) When you have become practised at this stretch, you can try this variation. Simply raise one leg straight out behind you, heel uppermost, until it is level with the trunk and arms. Do not point the toes and do not lift the hip of the raised leg. Try to keep both buttocks level.

7.2 For hamstrings (back of legs)

Stand facing a table of average height or other firm support, raise one leg and rest your heel on the table, stretching the whole leg to the sole of the foot. Both legs should be quite straight and the standing foot should point directly forward, so do not let it turn out to the side. The back should be straight and the two hips level, so you need to lower the hip of the raised leg. Then repeat with the other leg. If you cannot keep your legs and back straight, find a lower support. With practice, you will be able to raise the leg higher.

7.3 For hips and inner thighs

Lie on the floor with your buttocks touching a wall and your legs resting vertically against it. Your whole back from neck to tail-bone should be flat on the floor. Spread your legs apart as wide as they will go, keeping your knees straight. Keep the centre back of the heels and the back of the knees against the wall, and stretch the inner legs so that the insteps extend away from you. At the same time release the muscles where you feel it pulling, and let gravity help to stretch the legs nearer to the floor. Bend the knees and rest the feet flat on the wall for a few moments before sitting up.

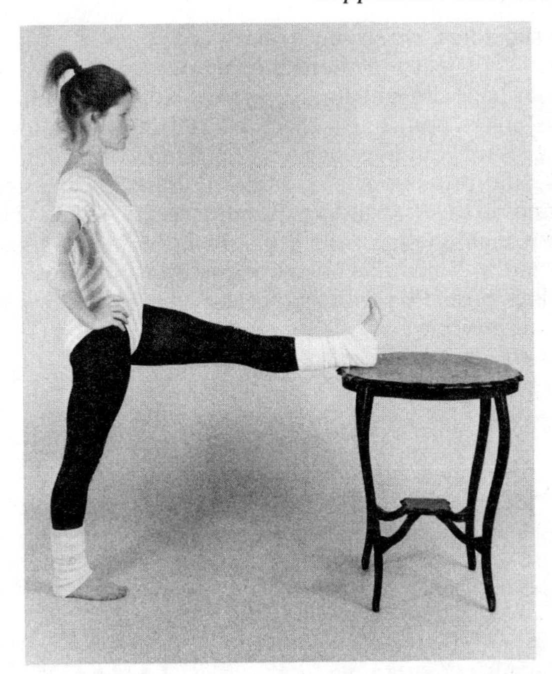

Exercise 7.2

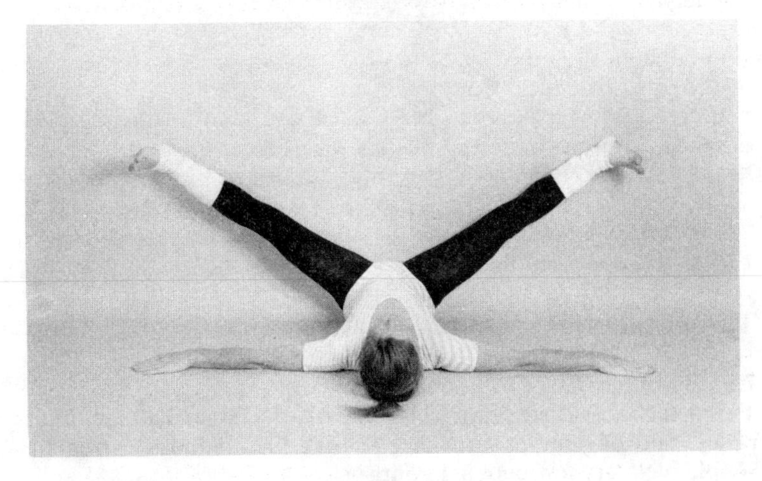

Exercise 7.3

7.4 For shoulders, wrists, upper back and chest

Stand with your feet together, and join the palms of your hands behind your back, fingers pointing down. Now turn your wrists, so that your fingers point in to the back and then up, moving your hands as high up your back as possible. Keep your shoulders down and back, and press your elbows firmly back, feeling your chest opening and rib cage expanding. Breathe deeply. When you can get your hands high enough, squeeze your little fingers between the shoulderblades. When this begins to come easily, you can practise the standing pose Prasarita Padottanasana (page 137) with the hands in this position.

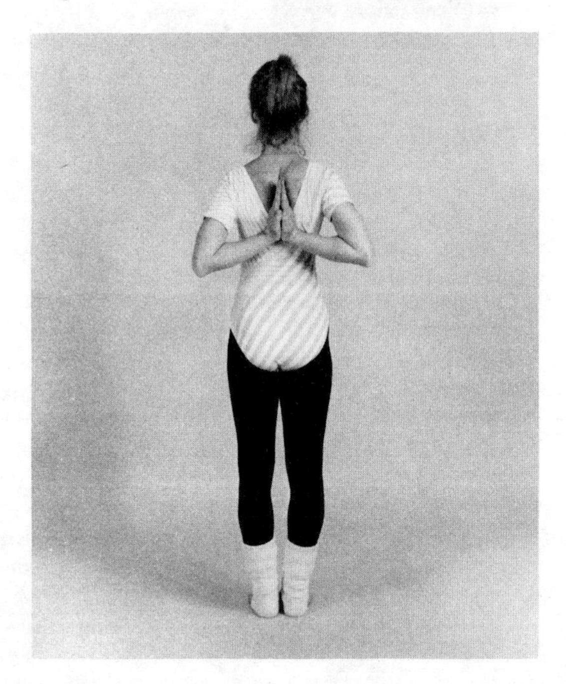

The postures

7.5 Mountain Pose (Tadasana)

This is the most basic of the classic poses, the basis of all the other poses, and of your posture in everyday life. It looks extremely simple, yet very few people in our society know how to stand well. To stand in Tadasana, place the feet together or hip-width apart, keeping them *parallel*. Feel how the weight is balanced on the feet, and try to distribute the weight evenly between one foot and the other, and between toes and heels. Notice any tendency you may have to be off-centre. The centre of the heels should be firmly on the ground, along with the outer edge of the foot and the big toe joint, where the big toe joins the foot. The arch should lift from the floor and the toes should stretch forward lightly on the ground and spread out as much as possible. Try to bring the big toes in line with the inner edge of the foot, keeping a space between the big toe and the second toe. The nail of each toe should face the ceiling. A useful exercise for those whose toes have lost mobility is to tie a belt in a loop around each big toe. Using the resistance provided by the belt, spread the other toes away from the big toes.

The knees should be quite straight, the kneecaps pulled up by the thigh muscles, and the hollows in the backs of the knees filling out as the legs stretch. The tail bone should move down towards the floor, the front hip bones lifting slightly, so that the pelvis is in a neutral position, neither tilting forward nor back. (You can feel the position of the pelvis by placing the hands on the front and back hip bones.) When the pelvis is properly aligned, the lower back will neither slump back nor cave in. There is a natural curve in the lumbar spine which should not be exaggerated; the whole spine should feel as though it is being lengthened, stretching upwards from the tail-bone to the crown of the head.

The lower ribs should not jut forwards, but the whole upper body, front, back and sides, should lift evenly up from the hips. Lift the breastbone and top chest and keep the shoulders relaxed. The shoulders should feel as though they are falling away from the ears and widening apart from each other, with the arms hanging loosely from them. Feel the weight of the forearms pulling on the shoulders. The shoulderblade at the back has a triangular shape; the bottom point of the triangle should move down towards the ground. The back of the neck should be extended, as though a string attached to the crown of the head were lifting you upwards. The chin should be level and not jut forwards. The head should feel well balanced, as though floating freely above the shoulders. You can test any exaggerated curves in the spine by holding a pole against it, or by standing with your back against an outer corner where two walls meet. The *sacrum* (spine at the back of the pelvis) and the back of the head should be placed in contact with the pole or wall, and you can then feel with your hand if there are any large gaps between the support and your spine.

This basic pose has been described in some detail, because the underlying principles apply to every other posture.

Standing poses

These are all intended for the legs, hips and spine.

7.6 Triangle pose (Trikonasana)

Stand with the feet about three feet apart, so that the distance between the feet is about the same as the length of your legs. Turn the feet, so that the left foot turns in slightly and the right foot turns out 90 degrees. The heel of the right foot should be in line with the instep of the left. The whole right leg should rotate outwards with the foot, from the top of the thigh. Make sure that the knee is rotated more towards the little toe than the big toe. However, the left leg should not turn in with the foot, but should also rotate outwards from the hip. This has the effect of 'opening' the hips and is difficult for most people. The knees should be held firmly in the legs, and kept quite straight.

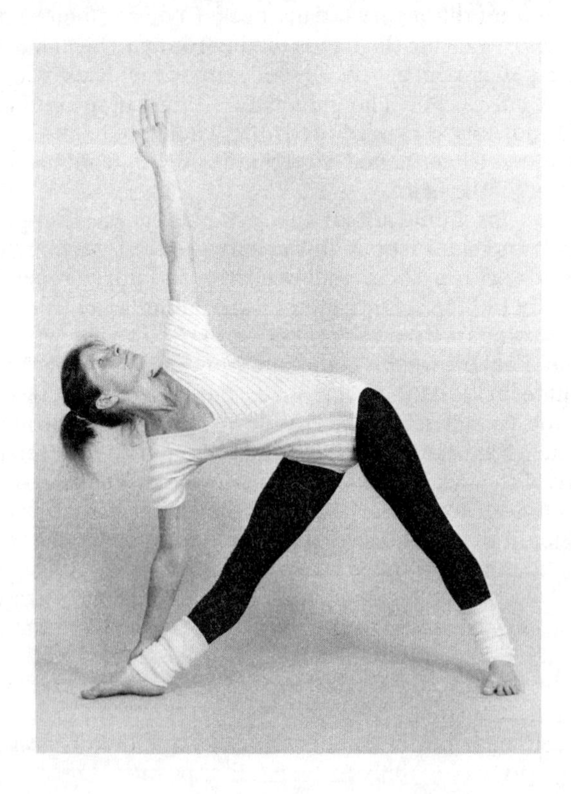

Raise the arms to shoulder level parallel to the floor, without lifting the shoulders, so there is plenty of space between the shoulders and the ears. On an exhalation, move both buttock bones to the left and stretch the whole upper body sideways to the right, lengthening as much as possible from the top of the right thigh to the right armpit. Then place the right hand lightly on the right leg, with the left arm stretching vertically upwards – both arms should move together as if one. If your right hand happens to touch the ground, you can rest it lightly behind the right foot, but *do not try* to get your hand to the ground. This is not a waist-bending exercise; the movement must come from the hips, so that the whole spine can eventually stretch horizontally from the hips to the crown of the head, parallel to the floor. If your hips are stiff and you try to reach the floor with your lower hand, you will only bend at the waist, and bring little or no benefit to the hips or spine. Keeping the back of the neck extended and the chin held in, turn your head and look up towards the upper hand. Keep the legs straight, the arches of the feet lifting and the thighs rotating outwards, hold the position for about twenty seconds with normal breathing, then return to your starting position on an inhalation. Repeat the pose to the left, reversing the directions.

7.7 Warrior pose (Virabhadrasana II)
Stand with your feet about four feet apart (the distance between them should be greater than your leg length). Turn the feet as for the Triangle pose, and raise the arms to shoulder level. The action of the legs and hips is exactly the same as in the Triangle. Bend the right knee by dropping the buttock bones towards the floor, keeping the tail-bone tucked in, until the knee is above the ankle, with the shin *vertical*. The knee must *not* roll forwards, so keep it pressing back. It is very difficult at first to keep the tail-bone in, the hips level and the bent knee back, but this must be worked on in order to bring more flexibility to the hips and enable the spine to stretch freely. The upper body should remain centred, leaning neither to the right nor to the left, and the whole spine should feel as if it grew upwards out of the pelvis. Practise in front of a mirror, or get someone to look at you to see if you are straight. You can turn the head to the right and look along the outstretched arm, but do not distort the position of the neck, or let the other arm drop lower than the shoulders.

Straighten the right leg, turn the feet and repeat to the left.

7.8 Side stretch (Parsvakonasana)

The Warrior can be extended to create a very powerful stretch in the whole trunk and the legs, stretching the inner thighs and the hip joints. From the position described above, stretch the upper body to the right, making sure that you do not disturb the position of the legs, and place the right hand or finger-tips lightly on the floor in front of the right foot. Extend the left arm alongside the left ear, palm down. Do not lean your weight onto the right hand, but carry the weight on your legs. Use the right arm to keep the knee pressing back, and against that resistance try to bring the right buttock bone forward and continue to rotate the left thigh *outwards* from the hip. Keep the tail-bone in. You should feel the hip joints being really stretched. Turn the upper side of the ribs and the upper shoulder back so that the breast bone turns towards the ceiling. If you cannot bring the right hand to the floor without disturbing the position of the legs or without turning the chest downwards, place a few books underneath the right hand. Eventually it should be possible to turn the head on its axis and look up towards the ceiling in front of the outstretched arm.

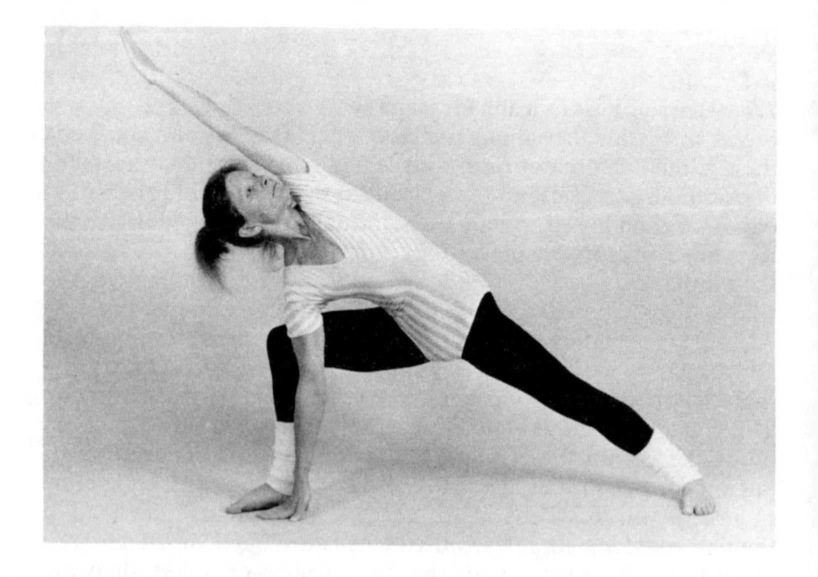

Breathe in as you straighten the right leg and stand upright, then repeat the pose on the left.

7.9 Reverse triangle (Parvirtta Trikonasana)
In this posture the upper body turns from the hips so that the chest and navel face backwards. The legs have to be strong and supple so that the pose can be held steadily while the spine stretches out freely from the hips. It is a good idea to practise the previous standing postures thoroughly before attempting this one, otherwise you will do the pose badly in the attempt to keep your balance.

Stand with the feet about three feet apart and turn the feet as for the Triangle (see p. 132), but make sure to turn the back foot a little further in towards the right, to enable the hips to turn more easily. Now swing the hips round so that you are facing backwards. Draw the right hip back as much as possible, and let the left hip move forward, dropping slightly towards the floor. Keep the legs absolutely straight and firm, taking special care that the back heel does not lift from the ground – it should stay 'glued' to the floor. The arms should swing round together as you turn, the left arm stretching down towards the floor and the right arm stretching vertically upwards.

If you cannot reach the ground with the left hand, place a low stool beside you to rest it on, or do the pose holding a block of wood in the left hand so that you can rest that on the floor instead (in other words, you are simply lengthening the arm by holding the block).

While holding the pose, keep the weight distributed evenly between the feet, and the knees firmly pressed back, and allow the spine to stretch horizontally from the pelvis to the crown of the head (as in the Triangle), opening the chest and flattening the upper back. Eventually, when the pose becomes steady, turn the head so as to look up towards the upper thumb. Inhale as you stand up facing forward, then repeat to the left.

7.10 Standing forward bend (Uttanasana)
This pose is used to stretch the hamstrings and spine gently, and also to rest the heart and lungs after doing the more strenuous standing postures. People with very stiff backs should rest their arms on a chair rather than allowing them to hang down unsupported.

Standing with the feet together or hip-width apart, turn the toes very slightly inwards. As you breathe out, bend forward *from the hips*, keeping the chest open, the spine extended and the head up, until you cannot stretch any further forward. Then relax the upper body completely, so that from the hips you are hanging down passively like a rag doll. Let the back, abdomen, ribs, shoulders, arms, neck and head become quite slack, so the head should hang

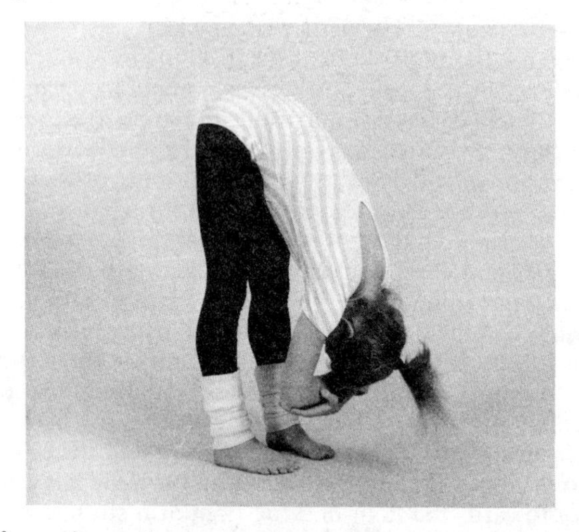

loosely from the neck. As you bend forwards, you should feel as though it is the action of lifting the buttock bones which causes you to bend. While you hold the position, breathing normally, continue to lift the buttock bones towards the ceiling and spread them apart from each other (try to do this, even if you can feel nothing moving at first). Release the muscles in the backs of the legs, following the powerful stretch that is imposed on them. Do not bend the knees. At first you may only be able to hold this pose comfortably for a very short time, but it will gradually become more relaxing.

To come up again, inhale, and *lift your head first.* Come up in one smooth movement, exactly as you went down, keeping the chest open, shoulders relaxed and spine extended, hinging only at the hips. Do not hunch the shoulders or bend at the waist.

Balancing poses

Several postures develop balance particularly, since they involve balancing the body's weight on one leg.

7.11 Half Moon (Ardha Chandrasana)

This is a good balancing posture, though when you first try it, it is better to practise with the back against a wall. Stand with your back against the wall and move into the Triangle pose, on the right side. Now bend the right knee, and gradually take the weight onto the right foot, lifting the left leg up sideways against the wall, and supporting yourself by resting the fingertips of the right hand lightly on the floor just in front of the right foot. If it is difficult to reach the ground, use a block (as suggested for the Reverse Triangle pose). It is very important in these balancing postures that the arch of the supporting foot is lifted well off the floor and that the knees remain straight. In this pose, the thigh of the supporting leg should rotate outwards (towards the wall), and the upper hip should turn back against the wall to open the hip joints. Both shoulders should touch the wall. By extending the raised leg firmly outwards (the sole of the foot should push away from you, do not point the toes) you can stretch the spine well in the opposite direction. Turn the head on the axis and look up towards the upper hand. The feeling of the pose should be light and exhilarating, like flying. Eventually you should practise the posture without the support of a wall.

To come out of the pose, bend the right knee and lower the left foot gently to the ground. Straighten the right leg, and breathe in as you stand upright.

7.12 Spread legs forward bend (Prasarita Padottanasana)

Attempt this pose only when you have gained some flexibility in the legs, hips and back, otherwise you will not really benefit from it. If you are stiff, continue to practise the basic stretches (pages 127–30) every day. This posture strengthens the feet and ankles, stretches the inner legs and extends the spine, 'ironing out' excessive curvatures, so that it is a good preparation for both forward bends and back bends.

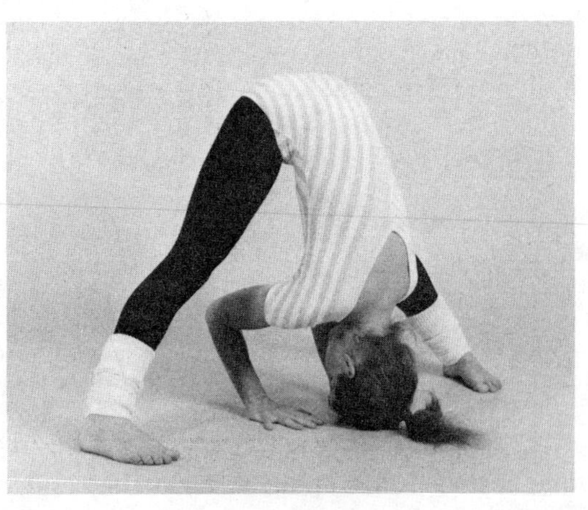

Stand with your feet parallel, about four feet apart. Make sure that your toes are not turned out, in fact you can turn them in slightly. Lift the arches and feel the firmness of the feet on the ground. Feel the inner legs stretching and stand very tall, with the pelvis level. Stretch the spine. Place the hands on the hips and bend forward *from the hips*, keeping the back straight; you will feel the pelvis rotating under the hands. Place the hands on the ground just in front of the feet, shoulder-width apart. If you cannot quite touch the ground without bending the knees, place the hands on a low stool or folded blanket.

Lift your head and look up, keeping the legs and arms quite straight. Spread the buttock bones apart, and allow the spine to stretch out away from the hips. The back should be straight, neither hollowing in nor humping up. Breathe normally.

For the second stage, continue to turn only from the hips. Exhaling, lower the whole trunk towards the ground, bending the elbows in, as if to try and bring your breastbone to the floor. If your head touches the floor easily, bring your feet closer together; you should have to stretch the spine thoroughly to bring the head down.

To come up, inhale and straighten the arms, then inhale again as you stand upright.

The Dog Pose (Svanasana)

There are two variations of this key pose, which can be practised separately or alternately in sequence. The first version described here (the head-down position) is basically a forward-bending movement, and the second (head-up version) is basically a back-bending position. Both poses strengthen the wrists and arms, and work the shoulders and upper back and chest, as well as stretching the legs and spine, so between them they stretch the whole body thoroughly.

7.13 Head-down position

Lie on your front, if possible lining the centre of the body up with a line on the floor, such as a join between floor boards. Tuck your toes under, keeping the feet hip-width apart. Place the palms of your hands flat on the ground beside your chest, spreading the fingers well, and making sure that the forefingers and thumbs are making firm contact with the floor.

On an exhalation, lift the whole body on the hands and feet, straightening the arms and keeping the legs straight, lifting the hips

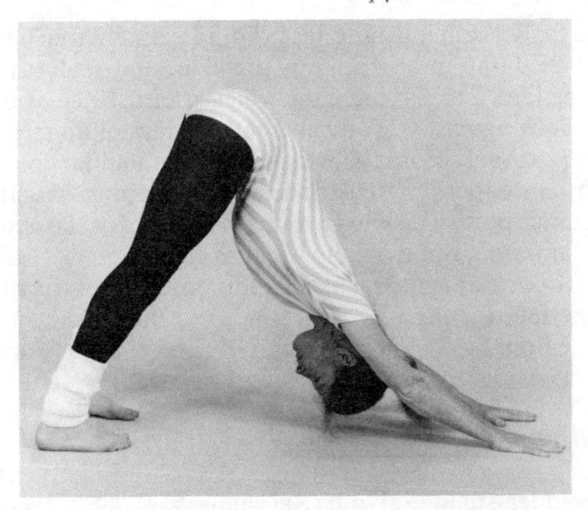

up and back, and dropping the head so that you look towards your feet. Press the balls of the feet firmly into the floor, lift the heels and lift the buttock bones up and back away from the head, until you can feel the arms stretching from the wrists to the shoulders, the shoulders flattening and the whole spine stretching from the shoulders to the tail-bone. Then try pressing the heels to the floor so that you feel a strong stretch in the backs of the legs. The heels probably will not touch the ground at first, and may not for some time. If the legs are very stiff, you can rest the heels on a thick book or on a skirting-board. Keep the head, neck and breathing relaxed all the time. Another variation which can be done by stiff people, or simply as a preparatory exercise, is to place the hands on the seat of a chair which is secure against a wall. This helps to stretch the lower back better if the hips and legs are stiff. To relax after the pose, rest down on to your front or on your knees.

7.14 Head-up position

This pose is done with the hands and feet in the same position as the previous one, so it is possible to move smoothly from one position to the other by swinging the body to and fro, keeping only the hands and feet on the ground throughout.

When you first practise this pose, start from the face-down lying position, with your hands beside the chest and toes tucked under. It is useful to practise with the feet against the wall. With an inhalation, straighten your arms so that you lift the body clear of the ground, keeping the legs straight and letting the hips drop towards the floor. Only the hands and feet should actually touch the floor. Tuck the tail-bone in as firmly as possible, and really stretch the backs of the legs. This is where the wall is useful, since by stretching the heels back against it, you can keep the legs quite straight. The arms lift up strongly from the wrists, but the shoulders must not lift or hunch; instead the breastbone lifts, widening the chest and stretching the spine. The whole spine should feel as if it is stretching from the tail-bone, not from the waist. Keep the breathing relaxed. When you become more practised at this pose, you can do it with the tops of the feet resting on the ground, but the legs must still stay clear of the floor.

Inverted poses

7.15 Shoulder-stand (Salamba Sarvangasana)

This is one of the most important yoga postures. It has many benefits, due to the inverted position of the body and the chin lock which stimulates glands in the neck, especially the thyroid which plays an important part in controlling the body's metabolism. All the internal organs benefit from the reversed pull of gravity, circulation is improved and the pose has a soothing effect on the nerves. It is a good one to do in the evening before going to sleep, especially if you suffer from insomnia, or are feeling 'wound up' and over-stimulated. When the pose is done well, it stretches the spine beautifully, including the back of the neck; however, care must be taken to position the body very carefully before going up, so as to prevent strain on the neck. To begin with, stay in the pose for only one or two minutes, but with practice, when the upper back and shoulders become flexible enough to allow a perfectly straight posture, and when the back and neck become strong, the pose can be held for ten to twenty minutes.

Start by folding a blanket two or three times to form a smooth thick pad large enough to accommodate your shoulders, and upper arms. Place a chair behind the blanket, about two to three feet away. Lie down so that your shoulders are exactly in line with the smooth edge of the blanket and your head is on the floor. This is to ensure that the back of the neck is not over-stretched and squashed into the ground, keeping the natural slight curve in the cervical spine (back of the neck). It should be possible to insert a couple of fingers underneath the back of the neck when you are holding this pose.

With an exhalation, raise your legs, keeping them straight, until they are vertical. Keep your whole back, down to the tail-bone, flat on the floor. (If you are stiff this may be very difficult, but it is a good position to practise in itself, perhaps with the legs resting vertically against a wall.)

Exhaling again, swing your legs behind your head, lifting the whole back from the floor, and rest your feet on the chair behind your head. Now interlock your fingers behind your back and stretch your arms out along the floor, drawing the shoulders away from the ears and lifting as much of the back as possible away from the floor, even the shoulder blades, so that your chest moves nearer to your chin. This position is known as the Plough pose. Now support your back as near to the shoulder-blades as you can, gripping firmly with your thumbs and forefingers and keeping the elbows in (they will want to slide out). Exhaling, raise your legs from the chair, keeping the knees quite straight, until the whole body is vertical from shoulders to ankles.

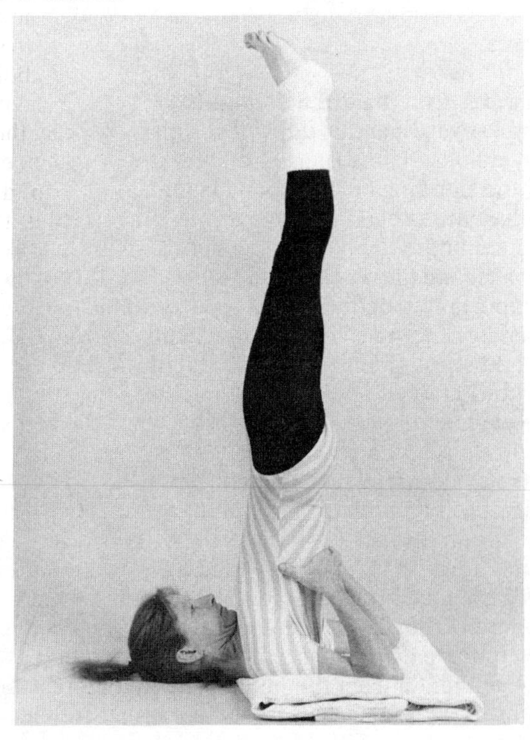

As you raise then lower the legs, the back should be disturbed as little as possible, so you should feel that you are hinging at the hips. If the back is weak, it will tend to collapse as you move the legs, or the hips will tend to move back to counter-balance the weight of the legs. As the back becomes stronger, make an effort to keep it straight, so that the hips are in line with the shoulders.

Throughout, keep the neck and throat relaxed, and maintain a steady rate of breathing. The chin should not feel jammed down into the chest, but the chest should move up to meet the chin. To come down from the pose, lower your feet about half-way down towards the chair, stretch your arms behind your back on the floor, with palms down, and gently roll your back onto the floor, one vertebra at a time. Lie on the floor and relax. If your back aches, draw your knees against your chest and hug them against you with your arms (better still, get someone to press down on your pulled-up knees for you).

Floor poses

7.16 Forward bend (Paschimottanasana)

This sitting forward bend is difficult for many people at first, as it requires very loose hamstrings and hips. It will come better after practising the standing forward bend (Uttanasana) and the Plough pose with feet on a chair. If you are stiff, practise this pose with a folded blanket under the back of the buttock bones, so as to tilt the pelvis forward, and use a belt looped around the feet to pull against. It is very important to understand the nature of the movement in the forward bends, otherwise you are more likely to strain the back than to loosen and strengthen it, so study the illustration carefully and note the rotation of the pelvis, which enables the spine to stretch forward evenly, and which is only possible when the hamstrings are able to stretch.

Sit up straight, making sure that you are balanced on the buttock bones and not rolling back with the tail-bone touching the floor. Pull the flesh of the buttocks back and out to the sides. Keeping the whole of the upper body straight, bend forward taking care not to hunch the shoulders. Hold your toes lightly, but if you cannot reach them without bending in the middle, use the looped belt around the feet. Using the grip on the toes or belt, stretch the front of the body, so it feels lengthened from the pubic bone to the breastbone. Fold forward only as far as you can without losing the stretch in the front

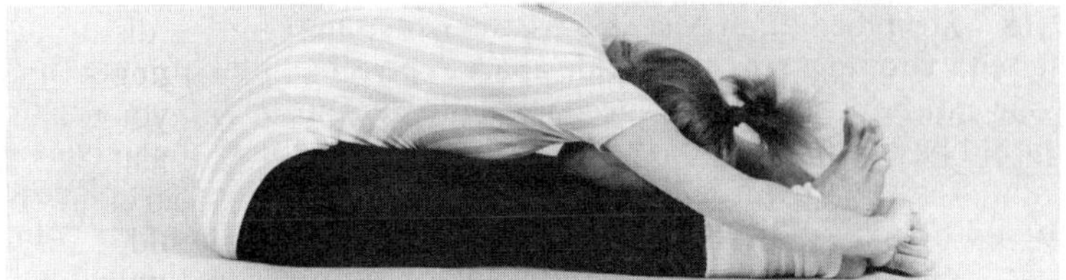
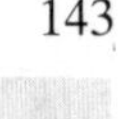

of the body and without bending the knees. Aim eventually to take the stomach and chest to the thighs before the head.

Keep the legs straight throughout, with the backs of the knees pressed to the floor, and the feet vertical and together.

7.17 Cobbler pose (Baddha Konasana)

Sit with the knees bent, so that the soles of the feet are joined in front of you, and with the back against a wall. Get the buttock bones right back against the wall and lift the spine so that the weight is taken entirely on the front part of the buttock bones. Keep the shoulders back and relaxed, with the chest lifted, and concentrate on relaxing the hips and thighs so that the knees can drop down towards the floor. You can rest your hands on your knees and press them down gently, but make sure that you *relax* under the pressure. Alternatively, you could place weights such as sand bags or heavy blankets on the knees.

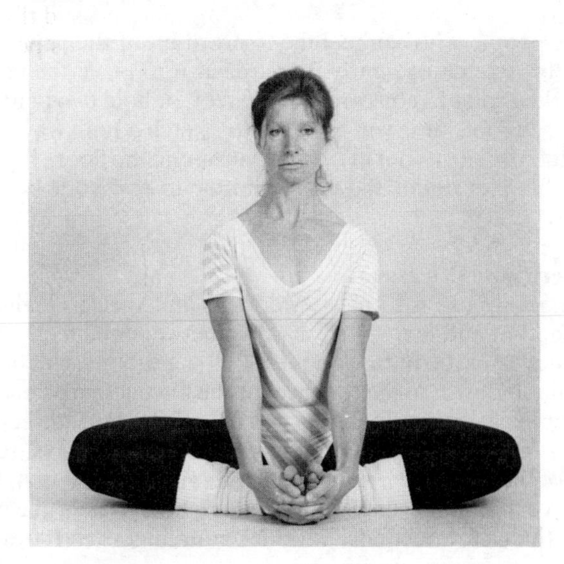

7.18 Stretched thigh pose (Upavistha Konasana)
Sit with your legs spread as wide apart as possible, making sure that your tail-bone is not rolling back onto the ground. The weight should be on the front of the buttock bones, enabling the pelvis to rotate slightly forward. This is very important; if necessary, place a folded blanket under the hips to raise them. Make sure that your knees are completely straight and facing up towards the ceiling. Stretch the soles of the feet firmly away from you, stretching the inner legs right down to the insteps. It helps to imagine that you are trying to sit on your thighs.

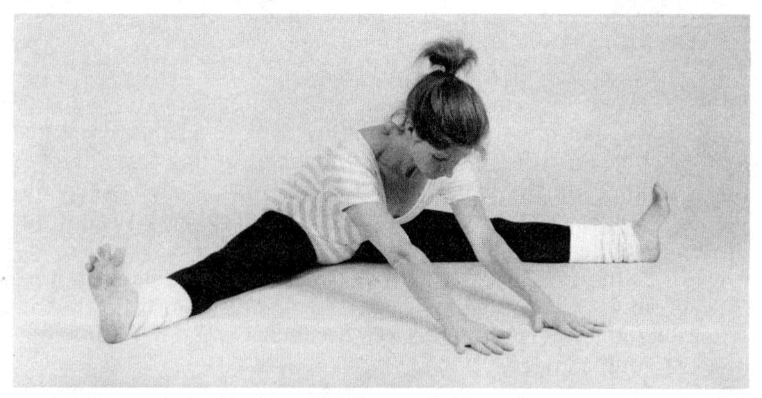

Supple people who can feel the forward tilt of the pelvis coming well can try stretching gently forwards as if to place the navel and chest on the ground. You can hold the feet, or hold two belts looped around each foot, or if you are able to stretch a long way forward, just stretch your arms out in front of you along the floor. Try placing a folded blanket under the chest and try to rest your breastbone against it.

7.19 Hero pose (Virasana)
This is a good pose for knees, tired legs and varicose veins. With knees together and feet apart, sit down between the feet, sitting on the outer edge of the buttock bones. Pull the calf muscles out to the side as you sit down, to make space for the knee joint to bend easily. If you cannot sit on the floor, place as many telephone directories as necessary under the hips. Do not turn the feet sideways, but keep the tops of the feet on the floor, even if this is painful at first. Sit with the back very straight, and, when you are able to hold the position for more than a few seconds, interlock your fingers and stretch your

arms above your head, turning the palms outwards. Alternate the interlock of the fingers so that you do not always have the same thumb nearer to you.

7.20 Twist (Marichyasana)

The twisting poses have a very soothing effect on the spine and can often relieve backache caused by stiff awkward posture. Once you are familiar with the principles of the twisting positions, you can use them at any time, for example while sitting at a desk, in the driving seat, and so on. The pose shown here gives quite an intense twist to the spine.

Fold a blanket several times or roll it up to form a thick pad. Place it about eighteen inches from the wall. Sit on the blanket with your back to the wall in such a way that the blanket is under the back of the buttocks, lifting the spine from the floor. Sit right on the front edge of the blanket, so that the pelvis tilts slightly forward rather than rolling back.

With your left leg stretched straight out in front, bend your right knee up in the air, drawing the right foot near to the right hip. With your left arm, hug your right knee, pressing the right foot firmly into the ground, and draw the whole spine upwards, sitting tall and 'opening' the chest. Now, with an exhalation, turn to the right and wedge your left elbow and upper arm against the outer side of the right knee. Place your right hand flat on the wall. Gradually twist further and further to the right, using the left arm pressing against

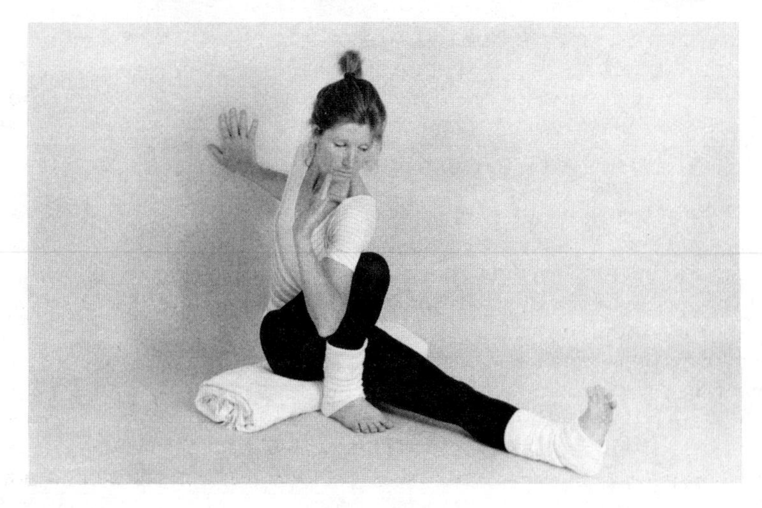

the knee and the right hand against the wall to help you turn. Do not let the right knee move across the body, but keep it upright. Also, keep stretching the spine upwards and keep the chest wide; do not slump or hunch the shoulders. Repeat the pose to the left.

Backbends

7.21 Kneeling backbend (Ustrasana)

When you first do this pose, practise it against a wall to make sure that you are doing it correctly. Kneel up with knees slightly apart and with the front hip bones touching the wall. The feet should be the same distance apart as the knees so that the lower legs are parallel. If you are stiff, tuck your toes under so as to raise your heels. Stretch the whole spine upwards, then, keeping your hips against the wall and your tail-bone well in, stretch back from the base of the spine, sliding your hands down the backs of your legs and then, if possible, catching your heels (keep your thumbs turned outwards). If you can catch your heels, let your head drop gently backwards and relax your neck. Hold for a short time, then inhale as you straighten up. Repeat two or three times, then sit on your heels and rest with your forehead on the floor.

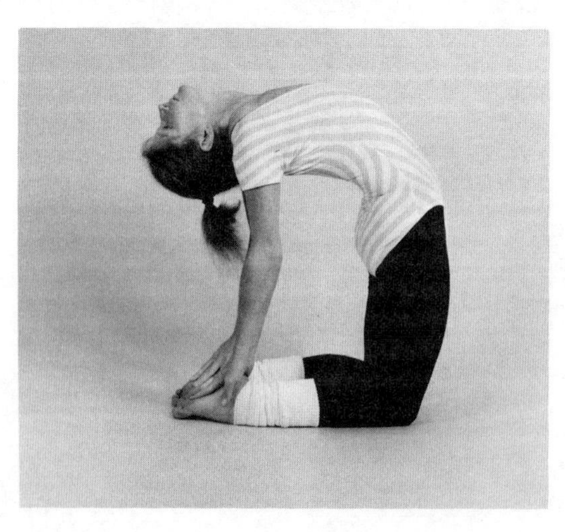

Lifting-up backbends

These positions are more strenuous to hold than the previous one, since they involve lifting yourself up off the ground. However, they should be done in as calm and relaxed a way as possible, without straining or holding the breath. Both start from lying face down on the floor.

7.22 Locust (Salabhasana)

Stretch your arms out in front of you along the floor, and keep your legs absolutely straight and together. On an exhalation, keeping the tail-bone tucked in, lift up your legs, arms, head and chest from the ground and hold for a few seconds with normal breathing. Try to stretch as much as possible, making the whole body longer.

7.23 Bow (Dhanurasana)

Bend your knees and reach back with your hands to catch your feet. If you are supple enough, catch hold of your ankles and flex the heels a little. Keeping the tail-bone in, exhale and lift your knees, thighs and chest from the floor. Stretch the back by pulling the feet with the hands and the hands with the feet. Relax and repeat two or three times.

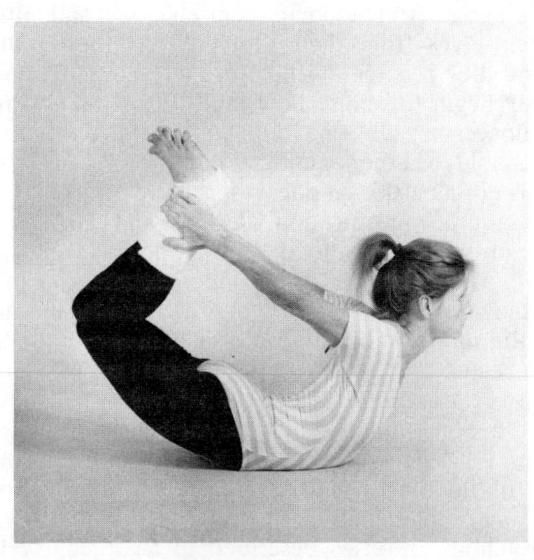

After doing the backbends, do a twisting pose to soothe the back, and then do a relaxing forward bend.

8

Relaxation

In the tradition of yoga, from which all the suppling exercises in Chapter 7 are taken, practice of the postures is always followed by a period of deep relaxation lying on the floor in a warm place in what is known as the *Corpse Pose*. It is one of the most important and difficult of the exercises, for it involves the letting go of all the activities and tensions that we are familiar with in our daily life, in order to be perfectly quiet in mind and body. When people first practise the pose, especially those who are habitually very tense, they find it a great effort to keep themselves still and impossible to detach themselves from their thoughts. As their practice progresses, and they become a little more relaxed and aware of their habits, they begin to realise how much effort they were wasting through unnecessary tension. Relaxation is the ability to let go, to loosen your hold, whether of muscles or of worries and desires. This letting go is not a battle – it does not require effort in that sense – but it does require concentration, alertness and clarity.

The person who is habitually tense, who is never still, always occupied, or always talking, or dependent on smoking or eating or drinking, may be generally aware that he is tense, but not able to recognise the *source* of his tension or its location in the body. It is difficult to realise that you carry a lot of tension in your hands or shoulders, for example, if you have forgotten what they feel like when relaxed. Sometimes the first real awareness of specific tension comes when it has become so chronic that it results in severe pain. Then a lot of 'undoing' has to take place, both through stretching and practising deep relaxation.

The stretching exercises described in Chapter 7 reveal each individual's areas of tension, and at the same time, they work on these areas by stretching and opening them. This practice brings an awareness which can be carried over into everyday life. Throughout the day, during all activities, you will become increasingly aware of your posture and body condition. A simple example is the way we hold our shoulders when doing something with the hands. Very often the shoulders are held tensely up and forward when they could easily be allowed to relax down and back without affecting what we are doing except to help it by releasing energy locked up in unnecessary muscular effort.

The stretching exercises are a very good preparation for deep relaxation. The stretching involved releases a lot of tension in the muscles and concentrates the mind. It is noticeable how much more easily and deeply the body relaxes after a good yoga or stretching session. If you were to lie down to relax in the middle of your normal activities, you would probably find it extremely difficult to concentrate and let go of the thoughts running through the mind. Vigorous exercise, while having the advantage of making you tired and possibly taking your mind off the day-to-day problems, does not necessarily stretch and loosen the body. So the best sequence is to take whatever hard exercise you prefer, then to do your stretching exercises, then to lie down and relax completely for about ten minutes. Yoga on its own, of course, should always be followed by the Corpse Pose.

Corpse Pose (Savasana)

Before you lie down, remove belts, glasses, contact lenses, hearing aids, and so on, and make sure that you are really warm, bearing in mind that you will be lying quite still on the floor for ten minutes or more. Spread a large blanket on the floor and lie down on your back with your knees bent up and your feet flat on the floor, feet and knees slightly apart. Let the small of the back relax into the floor and make sure that the tail-bone is tucked downwards towards the feet, lengthening the lumbar spine. As you relax this part of the spine it should flatten into the floor. When this has happened, stretch your legs out one after the other, and then let them relax. The legs should roll out from the hips with the feet flopping out sideways towards the ground. With your hands you can take hold of your head and pull it away from the shoulders in such a way that the back of the neck is stretched and the chin remains level with the bridge of the nose when you place the head back on the floor. If your chin sticks up in the air and you cannot keep it in, it means that the muscles in the back of the neck have become shortened, and the throat will not be relaxed. If the throat is tense the mind will not be quiet. In this case place a book or two under the back of the head so as to bring the chin in, and you will find that this is much more comfortable.

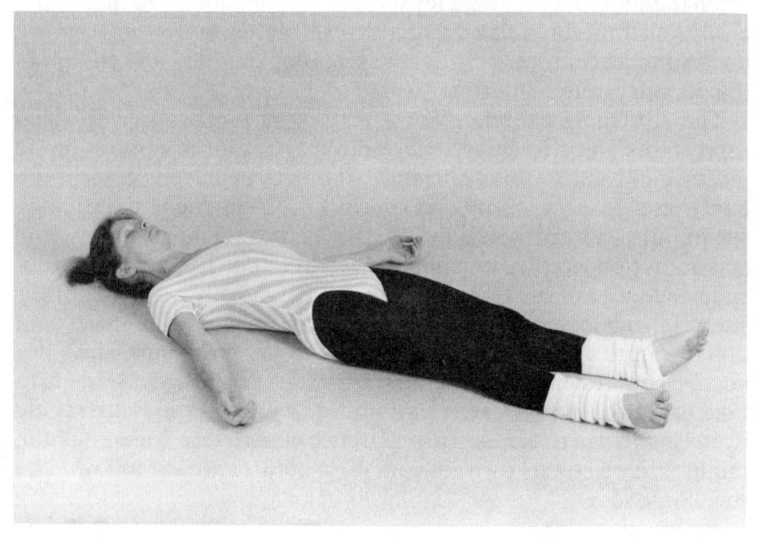

Corpse Pose

The head should be straight, with the bridge of the nose and centre of the chin in line with the breast-bone, navel and pubic bone. The weight on the buttocks should be even, and the legs should be an even distance from the centre line of the body. Stretch the arms out to the sides just far enough from the body to keep space between the upper arms and the ribcage. Rest the backs of the hands on the floor and relax the hands and wrists so that the fingers curl slightly in towards the palms. Move the shoulder-blades towards the feet, bringing the top of the shoulders nearer to the floor and rolling the skin from the collar bones towards the shoulder-blades. The breastbone will lift slightly, but the lower ribs should relax downwards and sideways towards the ground. Close your eyes and let the eyes relax, becoming heavy and dropping back into the skull, looking slightly downwards. Keep in mind the centre line of the body, from the top of the head to the heels, and imagine the two sides of the body falling away from that central line into the floor. Let the skin become soft over the entire body, including the scalp and the face, so that the skin of the face smooths out from the centre to the sides, broadening the forehead and space between the eyebrows, and broadening the cheeks and mouth, which should be soft at the corners. Relax the ears and the throat. Be aware of the back of the body pressing into the ground, as though the ground is moving up underneath you to support you, so no muscle has to work to keep you in position. Even the skeleton can relax.

Become aware of your breathing and notice how the breath has relaxed along with the body. The breath becomes very light, with quite a short inhalation and a longer exhalation; this pattern should not be imposed consciously, as it simply happens when the body becomes deeply relaxed. To help you still the mind, you can observe the breath, listening to its sound and rhythm, and concentrating on the slight pause between the end of the exhalation and the start of the inhalation. If it comes naturally, you can prolong that pause very slightly, but the emphasis should be on letting go rather than controlling. Thoughts will continue to surface in the mind, but they should be noticed and let pass, provoking no reaction. Whenever you notice the mind wandering away from the present moment, do not become impatient but cultivate the role of passive observer. So do not react, simply watch. Or if you do react, observe your reactions, so there is always a part of you which is unaffected by the thoughts, as by any outside noises or other external stimuli. The mind becomes passive, yet extremely alert. At first some people fall asleep in Savasana. This is not the aim and should not be encouraged; the mind should stay attentive and not drift away.

Problems with relaxing

Sometimes people find it difficult to relax on the floor because of stiffness and tension in various parts of the body. If the neck and shoulders are stiff, place a book under the head as described above. Often the lower back is tight and cannot relax into the floor. In this case it can be supported with a soft pillow or a folded blanket; ideally the space between the lumbar spine (in the lower back) and the floor should be very small. Alternatively, it is possible to relax flat on the floor with the lower legs, from feet to knees, supported on a chair or bed. This may well be the best way for people who get persistent backache when they lie down on the floor.

If the legs are very stiff, the feet could be spread a little wider until the back feels comfortable. Remember that as you practise the stretching postures, it will become easier for you to assume a relaxed position on the floor. Although it is best to avoid a totally unyielding surface such as concrete, one should never lie down for deep relaxation on a soft surface such as a bed. It is better to spread a blanket on the floor and use extra blankets or cushions for support where necessary.

If you are a rather tense person who becomes restless when lying still, you can try the relaxation technique of deliberately tensing and contracting each part of the body in turn, and then letting go, to experience the contrast between tension and relaxation. You could start with the feet and ankles and work your way systematically upwards. You will probably find that certain parts of the body are more difficult to relax than others, so spend more time concentrating on these areas.

If possible, you can place weights on certain parts of the body to help relaxation, for example on the thighs, lower legs, hands or abdomen (to ease backache). The eyes can be helped to relax by covering them with a soft weight such as a cloth tube loosely filled with rice. Generally the face and throat are the most difficult areas to relax, so make sure that you are not under a bright light, using the rice bag on the eyes if desired, and that there are not likely to be any sudden jarring noises (e.g. take the telephone off the hook). Relax the ears, directing them inwards rather than outwards. Relax the tongue to its very root so that it does not press against the top of the mouth, and make sure that the teeth are not clenched, or even touching. With practice you will find it becomes easier to relax the framework of the body, and will then be able to concentrate on finer points, detaching yourself more and more from the outside world, and from the ceaseless activity of the brain. It is as if you are retreating and shrinking away from the surface of yourself towards a deep and still centre, from which it takes you a little while to return to the external world.

There are some who are so tense that they have forgotten the actual feeling of being relaxed. They try to relax by various methods, but get nowhere, as they have no standard by which to relax. One method in such cases is to re-experience deep relaxation by exhausting the body till it can neither fidget nor even register how tired it is. When the body is well and truly exhausted it is allowed to relax, and in subsequent relaxation periods the feeling experienced at this moment is recalled. The body can be exhausted by long hours of physical work, or little or no sleep. In the army, for example, soldiers frequently stay awake all night on guard, work through the next day, then go to sleep early in the evening. Relaxing and falling asleep at such times is extremely easy and pleasant. In some eastern religious traditions, monks stay awake for five or more days and report the inner agitations dying down after a few days. Losing sleep is not particularly harmful once in a while, and can be useful in recapturing the true feeling of relaxation.

Another method for the very tense is to lie very still for very long periods. For a long time there is the internal need to move, but if it is not expressed, it eventually dies away. Once the need to move has gone, the person becomes aware of how much effort it costs to keep fidgeting. Whereas before it was an effort to keep still, now it is realised how much effort it is to move and the need to move can easily be conquered. Another, more recent, method of relaxation is to use bio-feedback machines. These register tension electronically and give you something to work against other than your own subjective feelings.

Coming out of relaxation

When you are ready to finish your relaxation, in the Corpse Pose or with any of the other methods, come back to life very gradually. The body, senses and mind need a little time to readapt to outside stimuli, and to return from a passive state to an active one. So first of all open your eyes softly, without focusing them to begin with, as though looking out from the back of your head. Just lie on the floor for a few moments, perfectly still, gradually bringing the eyes into focus and observing exactly how you feel – probably more relaxed than while you were concentrating in the Corpse Pose. If you are completely relaxed, you should impress this feeling on the mind before moving again. Then take a few deep breaths, and roll on to one side. Stay there for a few more seconds before getting up.

Meditation

Meditation is a practice associated with most of the religions of the East, although it has its Western spiritual counterparts. In Buddhism it is said to be 'one of the legs of the tripod that supports the religion', the other two being Wisdom and the Precepts. There are many forms of meditation, but most are essentially 'sitting' methods.

Apart from the spiritual aspects of meditation, there are many notable benefits. Practitioners are calm, energetic, and free of stress, insomnia, anxiety and neuroses. Probably most who meditate are interested in the spiritual aspects, although a growing number of practitioners do it as a calming and stress-reducing practice.

Physiological studies made of Zen priests with as much as thirty years experience of meditation have shown remarkable bodily changes during meditation. Electrical activity of the brain slows down, though it remains fully aware. The rate of breathing slows down to as little as four breaths (in and out) per minute, with abdominal breathing taking over from thoracic breathing. Muscle contraction intervals grow longer and longer although, interestingly, the pulse rate accelerates somewhat. Energy metabolism drops to 75 to 95 per cent of normal basic metabolism. In brief, meditation is a state of extreme stillness and relaxation, but full mental awareness. It is as if the meditator's body (and mind) is in the deepest of sleeps, yet he is fully alert.

In contrast to normal methods of relaxation, meditation works from the head. That is to say, apart from settling into a correct posture, the body is ignored, and the practitioner concentrates on the mental processes. Adopting the correct posture stills the breathing, which stills the mind, which in turn stills the body, and so on. Eventually, body and breathing awareness is left behind and the practitioner sits in the stillness of his mind. Most meditation-based religions do not distinguish between body and mind, and state that the two are one.

In theory, the technique of sitting in meditation is simple. The practitioner sits so that he forms a stable, balanced cone or pyramid-like shape. In this position the body consumes least energy. The traditional meditation posture is the full Lotus pose, where the legs are crossed so that the right foot rests on the left thigh, and the left foot on the right thigh. This is difficult for most people although it can be achieved with practice. The simplest method is just to cross the legs, or perhaps to sit Japanese-style – sitting on the feet. Whatever position is used, it must be balanced and symmetrical, and sustainable for half an hour or more.

First of all, fold a blanket to form a comfortable base, about three feet (1 metre) square. It is not possible to sit flat on the floor for any length of time without feeling some strain in the back or hips, so it is necessary to wedge some thick cushions under the buttocks. Some experimentation will be required to find the right thickness. Once you find it, it should immediately feel comfortable, and you should feel wedged into position, with your back held straight and your

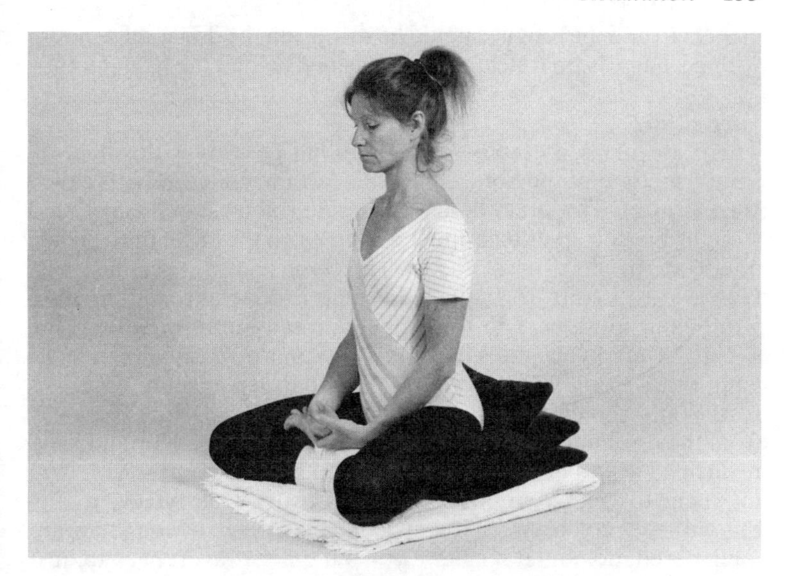

Meditation posture

weight evenly spread between the knees and buttocks. Choose a quiet spot in which to sit, with the light source behind you. The room should be neither too light nor too dark – it helps to sit facing a wall. If it has symmetrical patterning on, this will help you to sit straight. If possible, select a vertical line that faces you centrally, and then select a mark on it at which to gaze. This will help 'centre' you. Choose a spot where you will not be interrupted. Lock the door, or tell anyone in the house that you are going to meditate and that you do not want to be interrupted. Do not keep your meditation secret, or you will feel jumpy and nervous of being discovered.

Having sat down and wedged yourself into position, rock from side to side and from front to back a few times to find your centrally balanced position, and try to keep the body still thereafter. Loosen any restricting clothing, especially round the waist (such as a belt). The hands should hold each other and rest in the lap, as the arms will start to ache if they are allowed to hang down from the shoulders. Once more or less in position, straighten the back, drop the shoulders out and down (do not hunch forward), flatten the back of the neck, and pull the chin in slightly. Hold the head as if you were looking straight ahead, then drop the eyes to look down at an angle parallel with the slope of your nose. The jaws should be very lightly clenched, and the tongue should be resting on the floor of the mouth with perhaps its tip touching the gums just behind the front teeth.

'Just sitting'

There are many methods of meditation. To start with, the very simple method of the Soto Zen sect is recommended. This is called 'Just sitting'. The practitioner sits comfortably, cross-legged and straight-backed, eyes half open, gazing down the angle of the nose, either at the floor or at the wall if close enough, and just sits. However, 'just sitting' implies that that is done and nothing else. Bring your awareness to the immediate sensations of sitting, the sounds around you, the silence in between the sounds, the feel of your buttocks and knees on the floor, and the spot where your eyes rest. While you do this, thoughts will arise that will drag you away from the present moment and place. Just let them pass by and keep reverting back to 'just sitting' (and nothing else). To start with, you may need to check your posture every once in a while but eventually this will not be necessary. If you do have to move, or cough, or are interrupted, do not let it agitate you but quietly revert back to 'just sitting'. Many meditation schools recommend breathing practices during meditation, such as slowly counting the breaths and lengthening the out-breath. However, those with disordered breathing and tense stomachs may find that this merely makes them worse.

The early experiences of meditation are not startling. It will take some time to develop a comfortable sitting posture without back strain. As the habit of sitting develops, it will become extremely comfortable and effortless. Once the habit of correct sitting is acquired, you will notice how quickly the breathing starts to slow and settle down. Eventually it will become so fine that you should not be aware of it. Often you will notice many fluttering sensations in the body. These are habitual muscular tensions loosening off and dying away. Later on you may become aware of areas of deep tension in the stomach, back, neck, face or scalp. Eventually these will die away, and you may experience how certain mental experiences (not thoughts, but something like emotional colouring) die away with them. After some practice you will be able to sit completely still, alert and 'cool-headed'.

For some time you may not experience much at all. Certainly you must not expect any new or higher planes of consciousness, or an earth-shaking mental experience. If you are 'expecting' you cannot be 'just sitting'. With time, you will find the sitting sessions refreshing and necessary as an antidote to the stresses and strains of daily life. The experience of real stillness will act as a brake on other activities that tend to plunge you into mental turmoil.

As you get used to meditation you may find yourself sitting in absolute stillness for periods of up to an hour or more. If at any time the meditation makes you heady or aggravates any bodily tensions, give it up for a few days. Some may find that they can only sit once every four or five days, while others can do it every day. Try to sit early in the day, and when you feel well and your usual self.

9

All-round Fitness

Some of you are probably aiming for all-round fitness. Bearing in mind the different components of fitness this is obviously a time-consuming business. However, for those with the time and the inclination, a programme is given in this chapter.

Background to fitness

Before going into the programme in detail, it is essential to consider some of the background aspects of fitness. Exercise of any sort requires adequate food and rest.

Food

A large expenditure of energy in exercise demands a large intake of energy in food. For the average person with moderate fitness goals, this does not matter too much, as exercise will increase the appetite and sufficient food will be eaten. However, there are dangers for those who are undertaking a fitness programme to lose weight and so restrict their diet at the same time. It is not uncommon for such people to start to feel dizzy or sick during exercise. Do not combine a large increase in activity with a sharp decrease in food intake or you will suffer for it.

Many athletes also fail to understand the importance of food. They do an enormous amount of training, but somehow their bodies and performances fail to show the results. This is often due to insufficient food or eating too much junk food. Food of the right quality is especially important for athletes such as boxers who compete in weight categories and constantly have to keep a check on their weight. Without the right food you will make no progress in training.

Exercise is a *catabolic* or breaking-down process. During the subsequent rest period the *anabolic* or building-up process takes place. Without food and rest no building-up will occur.

Rest

There are two aspects to rest. Firstly an exercise programme cannot take place against a background of long, unremitting work. The body has only so much energy, and if this is mostly used up with a hard day's work, the exercise itself will be unpleasant and the anabolic process will not be able to take place. Of course the work itself might provide sufficient exercise, but this is unlikely. Probably the work will contain little or no aerobic activity or stretching, and its net effect will merely be exhaustion. In such a case the total amount of work will have to be reduced. It is probably safe to say that the real reason why the majority of people are unfit is that they have no time to be fit – work consumes most of their time. Reducing work time poses many problems, however health and fitness are of major importance, and time must be found for them.

The other aspect to rest is sleep. A physical life demands a good night's sleep. Exercise will help you to sleep, but late nights will not help your exercise. For those who tend to sleep badly, I suggest getting up early. This is not because early rising is proverbially good for you, but because it is the best way to regulate the pattern of your sleep. After a bad night's sleep most people linger in bed as long as possible, trying to make up for their missed sleep in fitful dozing which is of doubtful use. Instead of this fitful dozing, get up early. You will feel much the same during the day, but will find it a lot easier to go to bed and sleep well in the evening. A better sleeping pattern will gradually assert itself.

The fitness programme

A total fitness programme consists of work in several areas already mentioned. They are: strength, strength-endurance, stamina, speed, suppleness, and relaxation. To this one could perhaps add other components, such as agility and coordination. These are not strictly fitness components, but anyone who plays squash or similar games will appreciate their importance. Uncoordinated movement is inefficient movement which uses up more energy than is necessary. Fortunately two or more components can be combined in one workout. In the following abbreviated all-round fitness programme strength and strength-endurance; stamina and speed; and suppleness, relaxation and agility are grouped together.

Strength and strength-endurance

This section of the programme requires the use of weights or access to a gymnasium. The routine comprises five exercises which are all fundamental and essential weight-training exercises and cover the main muscle groups of the body. For a description of the exercises refer to Chapter 5.

1 Clean to chest (p. 75)
2 Bench press (p. 55)
3 Bent-over rowing (p. 58)
4 Incline sit-ups (with weight behind head) (p. 71)
5 Squat (p. 72)

When combining strength and strength-endurance in one work-out, tackle the exercises in the following manner. First do each exercise a dozen times with a very light weight. This is by way of a warm-up. Then do two sets of each exercise at 6 repetitions maximum (RM) (see p. 47) and take a rest between and after the sets. Then remove 20 per cent of the weight from the bar and do 15 reps-maximum, remove another 20 per cent and without a rest do 20 reps-maximum. If 100 lbs is your 6RM weight, then the routine per exercise would be:

12 warm-up movements
6RM × 100 lbs
Rest
6RM × 100 lbs
Rest
15RM × 80 lbs
20RM × 60 lbs

The first two sets work on maximum strength and the last two work on strength-endurance, which is why there is no rest between them. Some thought is needed in loading the bar to start with. Put on a number of smaller discs so that the removal of 20 per cent each time can be swiftly and accurately done.

Stamina and speed

Strength work is limited by the fact that you work to a maximum each time, which can quickly be exhausting. With stamina work, however, it is possible to go on for hours. As was suggested earlier, continue any type of stamina activity, such as running, swimming, cycling, skipping, using an exercise bike, and so on, for as long as it feels good. After a time a training period will establish itself. It might be that twenty minutes to half an hour each time will feel just right. Twice a week is the minimum, however (refer to the spacing of the sessions during the week). At some point in each session, when you are properly warmed-up and well into your fitness programme, put in some work at maximum speed. Go all out, and stretch and work every muscle in the body to the full. It is unlikely that you will be able to do much more than about ten seconds per burst, or more than about four or five bursts per session, since these all-out bursts are very exhausting. The gains you make from your strength work will help your speed work, and this in turn will help the stamina work. All aspects of fitness are interrelated.

Suppleness, relaxation and agility

For a full description of the stretching and balancing exercises in the following abbreviated programme for suppleness, refer to Chapter 7. These eight exercises will not take long to do, although the time you spend in each pose can be lengthened, as can the relation in the Corpse Pose at the end. Again, be careful not to strain yourself if you are stiff.

1. Triangle Pose (Trikonasana) (p. 132)
2. Dog Pose (Svanasana) (p. 138)
3. Seated forward bend (Paschimottanasana) (p. 142)
4. Seated twist (Marichyasana) (p. 145)
5. Shoulderstand (Salamba Sarvangasana) (p. 140)
6. Plough (Halasana) (p. 141)
7. Kneeling backbend (Ustrasana) (p. 146)
8. Half Moon (Ardha Chandrasana) (p. 136)

Finish off the session with the Corpse Pose, held for several minutes.

A complete agility session could only be gained by going to an acrobatic, trampolining or Olympic gymnastics class with specialist equipment and tuition. However, a very simple agility workout can be based on the following three movements: forward roll, cartwheel and handstand. Practise them on a soft landing area.

The forward roll is a simple head-over-heels to the front, rolling down the back. Do it first from a crouch position, close to the ground, and take care to tuck your head well in underneath as you roll forward. Gradually begin the move standing higher and higher, until it can be done from a full standing position with a roll back up on to the feet.

The cartwheel is a wheel movement to the side, balancing first on one straight arm then on the other, as the legs wheel over the top and back to the standing position. The action of the body with straight arms and legs spread wide is just like a cartwheel turning round. Practise it wheeling either to the right or left.

The handstand is a balance on straight arms, with the trunk and legs held vertically above. This is strictly a balance, but various agility movements can be developed from it. One of these is to go up into the handstand, hold it for a second, then drop down into a forward roll. Alternatively, drop from the handstand into a back arch (you will need a supple back and assistance). Eventually it can be developed into a forward handspring or even a somersault.

The handstand can be practised first against a wall or in a corner for support. If possible, get tuition in these movements (for example, in evening classes).

A good way to spread the sessions covering the various components of fitness over the week is as follows:

Monday	Strength and strength-endurance
Tuesday	Stamina and speed
Wednesday	Suppleness, relaxation and agility
Thursday	Strength and strength-endurance
Friday	Stamina and speed
Saturday	Suppleness, relaxation and agility
Sunday	*Extra* stamina and speed session if desired

Some of these workouts will not take very long – however, you do not need to exhaust yourself every time you exercise in order to benefit.

10

Fitness for Sport

If you do not participate regularly in sport or athletics, you may feel that this chapter has little to offer you. However, increasing numbers of people are taking up sport either as part of their own fitness programme or for its own sake and it is well worth considering as a way of combining keep fit and social activity. This chapter will help the sportsperson of any level of ability who wishes to improve his or her fitness in order to improve his or her game, and also includes a section for those who want to use sport to improve their fitness.

In one respect, fitness training for a particular sport or track or field event is a much simpler business than for the average person seeking overall fitness. The athlete or coach knows what he has to 'fit' himself to, and that is winning. If his performances improve or if he wins, he knows that his training methods are right, and if he loses, they are wrong. Fitness for the athlete is simply being able to perform as well as, or better than, the other athletes. It does not necessarily mean having all-round fitness, since the marathon runner does not need much strength, and the weight-lifter does not need much endurance. Provided an athlete can fulfil the requirements of his event, he can otherwise be unhealthy and neurotic. This is not of course to say that he would not be a better athlete if he were healthy as well.

The difference between past and present training methods is that nowadays the components of performance are much more clearly defined. The descriptions of what actually happens in a sporting performance are more exact, and consequently the training becomes more accurate. In addition, the athletes are constantly extending the limits of performance in training and competition, whereas a few years ago concepts such as being 'burnt-out' were dominant, and so athletes did not push themselves to the limits.

Modern principles of training are not really any different from those of two thousand years ago. In Ancient Greece, Milo of Crotona who lifted a baby ox onto his shoulders everyday, and so was still able to do it when the animal was full-grown, was doing what we now call *progressive-overloading*. He knew that to become stronger he had to lift gradually more and more each day.

The runners in Ancient Greece knew that to improve their running, their training had to consist primarily of running practice. This principle is now known as *specificity*, and the idea is that 'like produces like'. Runners may once have done other things that they thought would improve their prowess – now modern athletes rarely train in a way that does not mirror part of their performance in some way. We have lost the idea of *transference* or believing that the strength of wrestling can be transferred to swimming, for example, and are now much more specific.

Sporting performance

There are two aspects of a sporting performance: skill (including tactics) and physical condition. Just as a superfit athlete who has no real skill in the sport will not reach the top, neither will the one with superb technique who is exhausted in five minutes. The two aspects are interdependent, and this chapter is mainly about the physical conditioning for sport.

The most specific thing you can do is to play the sport itself, and to play a lot of it. When you do this, your skill and physical condition will improve at the same time. Of course it is not enough simply to play the sport anyhow; you must be able to recognise faults and deficiencies so that they can be corrected. You can either look out for the faults yourself, or rely on a coach or a video aid. However, some athletes often feel the need to immerse themselves in their sport. Swimmers, for example, may do thousands of metres in training, even though their event is only 100 metres. When they do this, they are trying to immerse themselves so completely in the activity that the rhythm and coordination of their sport becomes completely unconscious or 'natural'. Such training is really a form of *skill training*. Although good physical conditioning can be acquired from such long bouts of training, more specific training is required for championship performance.

Skill

Although the most specific training for a sport is practising the sport itself, there are limiting factors. From the point of view of skill, the pressure of a match or just rarity of opportunity may limit the chances for developing the necessary skills. To acquire skill in a particular move it must be practised many times, so if you only have a chance to perform it four or five times in a match, it is obvious that progress will be slow. In this case, the particular movement must be taken out and practised in isolation many times in a skill training session. However, the movement must be tackled as if in a real situation, and not done as a lifeless imitation. Skill training which is not specific, that is to say, not exactly like the real thing, is a waste of time.

Physical condition

The ability to be skilful is very much dependent upon physical condition. If you are in good condition for the sport you then have the 'time' or 'room' to try, perfect, and perform the various moves. However, the physical conditioning acquired from just playing the game may not be enough. The excitement of a match may push you to new heights, but will not lead to a systematic improvement. It has been found that greater progress is made by isolating the physical requirements, such as endurance, and working on them individually. In this way it is possible to train beyond the requirements of the match, and an athlete can go in for an event lasting twenty minutes knowing that he is fully capable of doing it for twenty-five minutes if necessary. In this way, better and better performances are achieved, and the frontiers of sporting performance are continually extended.

Planning your training

When training for a sport, the first thing to do is to define the dimensions of it. These are: duration, distance, speed, force, posture, and skill.

Duration

Most sports are played for a particular length of time, over which the physical effort must be made. If, for example, your sport requires twenty minutes of movement, then your training periods should be twenty minutes long. If your sport involves bouts or matches spread over a longer period of time, then your training must match this requirement.

Distance

Another way to reproduce the conditions of your sport in training is to cover the same distances. If training for tennis, for example, it is easy to work out the distances that you run in a match and the number of times. Your training should then simply mimic this.

Speed

Most sports are not played at a uniform pace but consists of periods at varying speeds. Thus each sport has a pace or rhythm which must be mirrored in training. If your sport requires forty-five minutes of running, with sprints at frequent intervals, then the training runs should be the same. Since your speed in training must be the same as that of the sport, it is pointless to train for much longer periods than your sport, because the pace would almost certainly be slower.

Abrupt changes of speed or pace in a sport are very tiring. It takes a real effort of will to force the body to put on a spurt, especially as you become tired. When actually playing the sport, the conditions of the game force you to speed up as required, otherwise you lose. However, in training, similar conditions do not exist. There seems to be a law of training by which all training tends to be reduced to a uniform pace. This must be continuously resisted. Whatever type of conditioning you are doing, try to mirror the speed and pace of the event.

Force

In sport one tries to overcome an opposing force. This force may be direct opposition, such as in wrestling and judo, or may simply be the force of gravity, as in high jumping. In contact sports, the opposing force is the other person. In sports that use equipment, such as rowing, resistance is provided by the weight of the equipment that has to be moved. In most cases the amount of force required can be measured, and in training a similar force must be used, not just for short periods, but mirroring the duration and speed of the event.

The particular way force is exerted in the sport has to be looked at very carefully. There are many ways that a muscle exerts force in contraction (see page 12), and the training must copy the way the muscles contract in the sport. It is important to understand the distinctions between maximum strength, strength-endurance, power, static (holding) strength, and braking strength.

Force, duration and speed all interrelate. A game is played against a certain resistance, for a certain length of time and at a particular speed, and training has to reproduce these conditions. Strength training should always be for the duration and at the speed of the sport.

Pulse rate check One reasonably accurate way to see if your training matches the duration, force and speed requirements of your event is to compare your pulse rate when actually competing with that of training. During competition, when you have a chance, get someone to take a record of your pulse rate. Do this over a number of events to obtain a reliable figure, and then try to achieve the same in training.

Aerobic base Many athletes whose event is not primarily aerobic find it advantageous to have good aerobic fitness. An example of this is the weightlifter who needs very little endurance. Nevertheless, many go running, and find that it helps their performance. This may be because they feel fitter, or because the running makes a recreational break in their training. Alternatively, endurance may be needed for training, as the time spent in training on all the individual components of a sport may add up to many hours per week, and so a good aerobic base may be very helpful. Often the athletes may be ahead of the scientists in devising new training methods. As long as you know the reason for it (in this case, experimentation) it can be a good idea to try different training methods, even if not particularly specific, and see how they affect performance. The aerobic athlete could try strength training, for example.

Posture

Many sports, for example canoeing and fencing, are done in a particular body position. The body consists of several hundred muscles and the interplay of muscles in various movements and positions varies enormously. By training in the same posture, you make sure that the right muscles are used. An example of how different muscles are used in two versions of apparently the same movement can be seen in the curl in weight training (see page 64). Different muscles are used according to whether the hand grasping the dumb-bell is palm forwards, knuckles forwards, or side on.

Skill

Skill is not something which can be considered in isolation, as it is conditioned by the physical factors. Skill, of course, tries to negate these factors by catching the other player at the right moment and using as little force as possible; however, where the abilities of two players are similar, the exercise of skill becomes more important. The trend in sport seems to encourage working on strength and stamina at the expense of skill. The reason for this is probably that it is easier to work on conditioning than it is to work on skill. However, as more and more people learn to condition themselves properly for an event, so players will be forced to study skill and tactics if they want to continue winning. However, acquiring skill is much easier if you are in peak physical condition.

To develop skill in a sport, it is necessary to find a good coach who knows the sport thoroughly, and who can apply the principles of training to the skills. If in doubt about any particular training method, ask yourself which aspect of your sport this training *mirrors*.

Hitherto we have talked about training to match the requirements of the sport. In fact, you need to train slightly beyond the requirements. Some sports are open-ended in the sense that the winner is the fastest or the strongest, and the training is always seeking to go beyond previous limits. Other competitive sports do not require much strength or endurance, simply enough to beat the opponent. In that case you should aim to train from 10 to 20 per cent more than is strictly necessary.

Personal requirements

There are other factors affecting sporting performance. They are concentration, courage, clarity, suppleness and relaxation, and body composition. The first three are the mental requirements of a sport. These are not easily trainable, but if you are aware of them, they can be enhanced.

Concentration

Concentration is literally focusing on the event to the exclusion of all else. In a sporting event there are many distractions: the spectators, your team-mates, and the personal tension of putting yourself on trial. Your mind can become a hornet's nest of thoughts pulling in all directions. More often than not, the competition environment is very different from the training one, and so it is essential to get used to it. The more competitions you attend, the more familiar they will be, and the easier you will find it to concentrate on your performance. When you focus on the immediate objective, you must lose sight of the wider implications. For example, a golfer may have to play one shot that will win or lose the match. If he thinks about winning, his shot may suffer. Instead he must play the shot in isolation, and not think about the outcome. In such cases, relaxation and meditation methods may be of great advantage.

However, concentration is not an inflexible mental attitude. It does not mean fixing onto a particular method of winning and sticking to it regardless of the cost. A concentrated mind is fully aware of what the other person is doing, and reacts appropriately. It excludes unnecessary thoughts and chains of thoughts, especially moments of inattention and day-dreaming. Your full attention must be fixed from the start of an event to the very last moment.

Courage

Courage is an obvious necessity in most sports, especially the rough ones. The sports push you to your mental and physical limits, and there is often the danger of personal injury.

People seem to be born with varying amounts of courage, but there are ways to tackle the problem. The first is to ignore courage as a specific requirement altogether. That is to say, do not regard it as something which can be produced at will or at the coach's request. Instead of going in for a sporting event and saying to yourself 'be brave', you should train yourself so thoroughly for the event that you know you can cope with it easily. Train harder than anyone else, and that will give you the necessary dose of courage.

Another method is the military one. Some military units have 'confidence training' areas, which often involve doing dangerous things on high ropes. The soldiers are not given much time to think and become frightened but are propelled from one nerve-racking task to another. This kind of training eliminates hesitation and instils courage. Do not experiment with such methods on your own – get expert guidance. In a similar way, if your sport involves taking a particular risk, you will find that practice helps to make it less intimidating.

Clarity

Winning in sport is becoming a more and more complex process, especially as the rewards and publicity increase. The athlete needs to understand all the aspects of skill and conditioning of his game, as well as the rules and procedure, and perhaps most important of all, he must understand his own psychology. He should know where he is going, why he is going there, what he expects to find, what he is going to do afterwards, and so on. He should be able to look at his acts and achievements objectively, and not be misled by illusions.

More athletes fail because of some mental block or problem than from any other cause.

For example, you may win because the opposition was badly off form, or because the referee made a decision in your favour. The correct reaction to this is not self-congratulation, but the acknowledgment that you were lucky, and the resolve to keep training hard. Similarly, too many athletes look for excuses when they lose. These are always at hand; for example, blaming the referee or citing injuries. The correct reason for losing should be written down in your training records and something should be done about it. All this needs clarity and the ability to see what really happened and to admit it to yourself.

Suppleness and relaxation

In recent years athletes have paid more and more attention to developing suppleness and flexibility, for various reasons. Firstly, a supple body helps avoid injuries to the joints and muscles. It has more 'give' for the sudden moments of exertion. Secondly, a stiff body has a limited range of movement, whereas a supple body can do far more and has greater potential to develop skills. Finally, a supple body can move faster and exert more force. Try clenching your fist and tensing your arm, and seeing how fast you can make a punch. Then loosen the arm and fist, and make the same punch, tightening the fist only at the moment of impact. You will see that the latter is much faster. In addition, a tense body burns up more energy than a relaxed one, and prevents the blood from getting to the muscles. It is necessary to relax where possible during most sporting events or between games, so as to minimise energy consumption and circulate the blood to the working muscles. Whereas a well-stretched muscle can exert more force at the start of a contraction, in some skill movements a super-stretch may be a disadvantage. It is sometimes necessary to hold a position, and not bend all over the place. However, it is an advantage for most throwing or ballistic events. Methods of stretching and relaxation are described in detail in Chapter 7.

Body composition

The composition and size of your body is not really affected greatly by training. However, it is important to assess yourself to determine whether your body shape and size is right or wrong for your sport. It is not uncommon to see people persisting in a sport even though they are not built for it. That is up to the individual, but if progress is slow, it is time to be realistic, unless the game is being played at a very light-hearted level. To a large extent the sport itself sorts out the people with the right build for it, especially at the higher levels.

Weight Although (in general) a larger person can lift heavier weights, if you compare the weight lifted with body weight, a bigger person lifts less per pound bodyweight than a smaller person. A large person can move a larger external weight (or throw a lighter weight further) than a smaller person, but is not as good at throwing himself about, as in gymnastics, as a lighter person. That is not to say that he cannot do it, but that a smaller person can usually do it better. If a sport requires agility and dexterity, a heavy build may be a disadvantage. Greater strength per pound also gives the lighter person an advantage in events requiring endurance, as he carries his body more easily.

Height This is another factor affecting performance. High jumpers tend to be tall but light, with relatively long legs and short bodies. However, the high jumper has a high centre of gravity, which puts him at a disadvantage in body contact sports where balance and contact with the ground must be maintained. Shorter legs are more advantageous in abrupt turning movements, such as in soccer, and legs which have a proportionately shorter lower leg are an asset in jumping. Those with long arms will tend to be better at throwing.

Taking up a sport

Coaching

By far the most important stage from the point of view of skill and technique is the very beginning, when you are taught the rudiments of the sport. It is essential to get good instruction and coaching right from the start, as this is when it has the most impact – you will be approaching it with a fresh and eager mind. If you are taught correctly at this point it will be an enormous advantage; if you are taught incorrectly, eliminating bad habits will prove extremely difficult, if not impossible, later on. Look around for a good coach before you start.

Peaking

The main principle of conditioning is overloading, that is, gradually doing more and more. For various reasons, both psychological and physiological, it is impossible to sustain an ever-improving performance. Usually training has to follow cycles of greater and lesser intensity, although the general trend must be upwards. Over a year there may be an off-season and a preparatory and competition season, based round the calendar of sporting events. Even on a week-to-week or day-to-day basis, training may have to follow a rota of light, medium and hard sessions. This pattern may be an imposed one which you try to follow, or it may be determined by your mood, so that you push yourself hard when you feel good, and ease off when you feel tired.

One factor which is always fixed is the event itself. You must bring yourself to a sharp edge for the competition, so during the weeks just before it the training must get harder and harder, even though it is still following a pattern of light-to-hard sessions, and should reach a peak about a week before the event. You will know, or should find out, how long it takes to recover completely from a spell of hard training, and so should stop in time to enter the event feeling fresh and sharp.

Taking the long-term view, the period in life when an individual is capable of peak athletic performance is relatively short. If you are young and think you have some sporting talent, it is probably better to push yourself to your limit for that period, sustaining your improvement for as long as is humanly possible, then retire, whether you win or lose. A few athletes find it possible to reach new heights after a period of inactivity – occasioned perhaps by illness or injury – but most do not. Give yourself a period, say five years to train hard, and then move on if you have not achieved your goal.

Age

Peak physical condition is reached around the age of twenty-five. In some sports, such as swimming and gymnastics, the best physical performance is achieved much earlier, perhaps in the early teens. Many athletes can and do carry on past their physical prime, particularly in those sports where skill and experience can make up for a decline in physical abilities.

Bearing in mind the age at which the peak is reached in most sports, it is wise not to start your children in serious training too soon. The problem is one of motivation, that is, maintaining interest. An early start is necessary, but training hard for years on end is extremely difficult. Many ambitious parents start their children in a sport at the age of seven, only to find after five years or so (which is really quite a long time) that the child has lost interest.

Another problem with the early starter is the one of bridging the gap between childhood and adulthood. A young athlete may get quite good as a junior competitor, but then find the switch to the adult league too much for his pride, if he does not win to start with. Training can also interfere with social life, which is very important for teenagers.

It depends on the sport, of course, but serious involvement in a sport is often better left to the early teens, or even later. Parents should never attempt to force their own sporting interests onto their children, but let them follow their own inclinations.

Diet for the athlete

Athletes need a balanced diet in terms of calories and nutrients. When the calorie content has to be low, care should be taken that there is sufficient nourishment. For example, the jockey has to be careful that his diet is nutritionally sound bearing in mind the low food intake. A nutritional imbalance is not such a danger with larger consumptions of food. Food should be taken not less than two and a half hours before a competition or a match. The food is then completely digested, and blood needed for exercise is not diverted to digestion. A meal consisting mostly of carbohydrates (bread, spaghetti, and soon) will be digested more quickly than one consisting mostly of fats or proteins. Except where the event is more than an hour long, there is no need to take glucose drinks during exercise. Too much glucose can in fact be harmful. However, the fluid balance in the body should be maintained, and regular amounts of water should be taken to replace what has been lost. This will obviously vary according to the event, clothing and weather.

There is a danger that athletes participating in sports with weight categories may not develop normally, fail to reach their full potential, or become ill if they keep their weight down artificially. If you wish to keep your weight down you should observe certain precautions:

1 Get an expert using skin callipers to assess the percentage of body fat, and check it is not less than five per cent. If it is, medical clearance should be obtained.
2 Your diet should be medically approved.
3 Weight loss through sweating and fluid loss by using plastic suits, saunas, diuretics and so on, should be avoided, and you should aim to lose weight by following the correct diet.

For stop-start games such as football, a diet which is relatively high in carbohydrates should provide an adequate supply of glycogen in the muscle for best performance, if sufficient rest is taken between practices and matches. For longer, non-stop events, such as the marathon, performance can be improved by boosting the store of glycogen in the muscle before the race.

First the store of glycogen should be depleted with a very hard workout, then a diet low in carbohydrates should be followed for the next three days. However, a minimum of 60g of carbohydrates must be consumed on each of these three days. If exercise is taken during this period, the depletion of the glycogen will be increased. Next, switch to a high carbohydrate diet for another three days, with a minimum of physical activity. This should bring you to the competition with a large boost in muscle glycogen.

Points to watch

There are one or two pitfalls that the average sports enthusiast must beware. The first is the word 'training'. Ask somebody how they know they have trained well, and it is likely that they will say 'because I feel exhausted'. In other words, training is equated with exhaustion. In fact, training for a sport is done for one reason – to improve performance – so really the only good evaluation of training is whether the performance has been improved in some way or other. This means keeping training records. If you know that what you can do now is better than what you were capable of one year ago, or even one month ago, then you know that you are improving. If, in addition to this, you are successful at your sport, then you know that the training is right.

If you do not know what you were capable of a year or three months ago, you are probably marking time. Sport can attract the exacolic or workaholic, that is, those who just need to exhaust themselves in long training. Often such people do well at sport. However, to become a real champion requires thought and careful training methods.

The other pitfall is going blindly into a particular *type* of conditioning. For strength, most people naturally think of weight training and for endurance, running. However, it is just not good enough to push a few weights or go for the odd run. Both these training methods have to be carefully used and tailored to the event, otherwise they may even end up harming performance. Measure up your sport and train to those measurements.

Sport for fitness

Most of this chapter has been about getting fit for your sport. Many, however, may not want to jog or do exercises, but would prefer to play a sport or a game to improve their fitness. In this case there are a few points to note.

There are very few sports that train all the main fitness requirements. Apart from swimming, all sports tend to tighten the muscles and reduce suppleness. Many athletes are supple, but often that is because they do suppling exercises to improve their game. Most sports will make you fairly strong in the limbs, but not exceptionally strong, unless working against more than bodyweight. Since stamina is the main component of fitness, all the sports that require you to run around a lot, such as football, tennis, squash, hockey, and so on, are good for fitness. Most of these, however, are stop-start activities, and studies done measuring the amount of time spent in running during a football match for example show that a third or more of the time may be spent virtually standing still or walking. Obviously a lot depends on how hard you play and whether you are a forward or a back. It may be possible to get more exercise in a thirty-minute continuous run than in a ninety-minute football match. Sports that require bursts of fast activity, such as squash, may be dangerous to the not-so-fit or those over thirty-five. Such games require preparation and should be played regularly (two or three times per week), but certainly not only occasionally.

All the precautions that apply to exercising apply equally to playing sport. Build up to it gradually, warm and loosen up before you start, and at the end of the game do not stop abruptly, but gradually warm down. The fitness derived from any sport depends greatly on how hard you play which makes comparisons between various sports very difficult. However, just getting out into the fresh air or a different environment, using your body and doing something that is enjoyable will be good for you.

11

Fitness after Illness

Many people cannot even begin the simplest exercises recommended by keep-fit instructors and others. This may be due to illness or injury, with resulting loss of muscle strength, bulk and coordination. Sometimes the muscles have to be coaxed back into normal activity from a state of total weakness where the slightest movement is difficult. Usually such people are under the supervision of a doctor or physiotherapist. However, professionals have a very limited amount of time to spend on patients and the individual quickly has to do most of the work himself. Sometimes the reasons behind the various techniques are not explained to the patient, or they are not understood, and he may come to the conclusion that he can do better himself. In most cases this is unlikely. What follows is a brief explanation of some of the principles of rehabilitation; it is not a substitute for a trained helper.

Rehabilitation

When injured or ill, a person may respond subsequently by staying inactive or altering his normal physical patterns to compensate for a loss of function, for example, by developing a limp. Both responses must be avoided. Inactivity leads to increasing muscular waste and loss of coordination, and the changed patterns of movement may become so habitual that normal, efficient, balanced, full-range functions are not resumed.

In such cases the patient needs to recover his normal strength and muscle size and his normal movement as quickly as possible. Movement may be complex, such as walking, or fairly simple, such as getting an elbow joint back to normal after an operation. In the case of the elbow joint, not only must the affected muscles be retrained but the joint itself must regain its full range of mobility.

Muscle development

When the force a muscle can exert is extremely low, various means are available to make it stronger. The progression of treatment ranges from moving the muscle passively, helping it to move, making it do its own work, and finally making it work against resistance.

The environment in which muscle work takes place can be changed so as to modify the force of gravity and so reduce the resistance. This can be done by suspending a limb in a sling for example, so that the resulting movement is like that of a pendulum, or by suspension in water, or by sliding it along a slippery surface.

When the muscle is virtually incapable of movement, an external force is used to take it through the full range of movement. This is usually done by the physiotherapist, who props the patient in a suitable position and isolates the limb so that it alone will move. In the case of somebody who cannot move a leg, for example, the physiotherapist does it for him, simulating the exact movement, perhaps using a gravity-reducing aid such as a sling. The patient himself is passive, and the physiotherapist makes the limb move.

Eventually, as the muscle or limb gets stronger, the physiotherapist will only assist the movement where it is weakest. At this stage the patient is actively moving himself, with some help. Next, the physiotherapist may provide resistance, within the range of movement of which the patient is capable. This stage is a combination of resistance and assistance, and the helper needs to judge the muscle's capabilities very accurately.

Eventually the patient can move the muscle himself against the force of gravity. At this point the muscle is strengthened further by working against resistance. This can be managed by the therapist resisting the full movement or by the patient moving some external weight, either directly or by pulley. Usually the particular muscle movement is isolated, and pulleys and weights are placed for maximum effect.

This rehabilitation process helps to achieve a number of things. Firstly, if gradually strengthens the muscle; secondly, it helps the muscle return to correct movement patterns and the discarding of faulty ones; and thirdly, it prevents the forming of deposits which would hinder full muscle and joint movement.

Muscle stimulation

Control of the muscles is by way of the nervous system. The end organs of this system lie in the muscles, tendons and joints, and are called proprioceptors. These are stimulated by stretch and tension. However, stimulation must be above a certain level to have any effect.

The three methods of stretch, tension and sufficient stimulation are used in rehabilitation. Tension is provided by resistance in one form or another, such as gravity, the physiotherapist's hands, or weights. When a muscle is stretched, its reflex action is to contract. This is used in physiotherapy when the patient is first commanded to stretch, and then to pull in the opposite direction. Sufficient stimulation is achieved by using maximum effort and several repetitions. When the patient is able to make maximum effort, further progress can be made by bringing more related muscles into play.

Normal body movement is very rarely in a straight line. The action of lifting a cup to the lips, for example, involves a certain amount of circular movement. Normal movement is often in a diagonal or spiral, for example, when throwing a ball, and so the rehabilitation of a limb takes account of this. A leg which is being strengthened may be made to work along a straight line, but with a twisting action at the start or finish.

Various techniques are used to elicit maximum response. Sometimes the muscle is worked one way against resistance, then immediately back the other way, also against resistance. Also, a limb may be held at any point in its range of movement, and then made to maintain its position against rhythmical pushing and pulling. Sometimes a limb is held at a particular point in its range of movement, made to resist this maximally, then allowed to relax as the resistance is removed. The last two techniques help to extend the range of a limited movement.

The muscles may work in three ways: they may shorten against resistance, lengthen against resistance, or hold against resistance. The first can be seen in pushing or pulling a weight, the second in lowering a weight slowly to the floor, and the third in holding a weight in position.

The muscle is built up by gradually increasing the resistance, the speed, and the duration of the exercise. Progression does not necessarily involve all three. In muscle-lengthening work, one progression is to do the work more slowly. The muscle must not be overloaded, as this may prevent it from contracting, or even damage it, but on the other hand it must not be underloaded since this will not strengthen it (although it may prevent muscle wastage). Generally, exercises for strengthening are slow and accurate. As for duration, the aim is five minutes in every hour. It is not sufficient merely to do the exercises, as the manner in which they are done is most important. The patient must concentrate on the form and content of the exercises.

Once the muscles are built up, the patient progresses first to more skilled movement, perhaps using various games in the occupational therapy department, then gradually to his ordinary everyday activities or sport, taking care not to attempt strenuous activity too soon.

Body movement

Re-education of body movement may start in bed where the patient can only lie on his back. The patient should first learn how to roll over onto his side or front, then to prop himself up on his side or front (using the arms), and then to swing the legs over the bed and into a sitting position. From the bedside he can learn to descend to the floor and move around, crawling if necessary. From a sitting position the patient can learn to stand up, usually starting sitting between two parallel bars which are used to pull the body up and into a standing position. Once in the standing position, the limbs will gradually become accustomed to bearing weight and the patient gradually learns to walk freely and unaided. In the various stages of the progression from lying to walking, the patient also has to learn the reverse procedures such as sitting down, lying down, and rolling on to the back.

A considerable amount of skill and ingenuity is required to coax limbs back into normal habits. The correct positioning of pulleys and patient is also essential. Where possible, use proper equipment and follow the advice of trained people, such as physiotherapists.

Avoiding heart disease

One of the major spurs to the increase in physical activities in the last decade has been the incidence of death from heart diseases. At one point in the 1960s 55 per cent of all deaths in the United States were from heart disease.* Younger and younger people have been dying from heart attacks, and considerable research has been undertaken into the various problems of the heart. Causes and cures are not yet clearly defined, but several 'risk factors' are recognised,

* *Aerobics*, K. Cooper.

and many of them can be reduced by the ordinary person. Neglect of exercise and diet are two key elements which can be recognised in the risk factors in the following list:

1 Obesity
2 Hyperlipidemia (high fat level in blood)
3 Hypertension (high blood pressure)
4 Smoking (cigarettes)
5 Physical inactivity
6 Psychological and social stress
7 Certain diseases (e.g. Diabetes mellitus)
8 Heredity

To help prevent coronary disease, it makes sense to eat less generally, reduce the intake of animal fats, give up smoking, and take more exercise. You can do nothing about heredity, although if there is a history of heart problems in your family, there is no reason why you should not try to minimise the chances of being affected. Psychological and social stress can be reduced, though some very fundamental changes in lifestyle and outlook are necessary, and by no means easy to achieve.

It is particularly interesting how many of the risk factors interrelate; many of them are all part of the same parcel. For example, obesity may be the result of inactivity or stress, and it in turn contributes towards high blood pressure. The trick is to break the vicious circle, and exercise seems to be one of the best ways to do it. However, exercise in its widest sense is necessary, not just increased physical activity. If meditation and relaxation are included in an exercise programme, they will help with stress problems. Whereas the link between heart disease and the inactive, heavy smoker seems fairly obvious, it may not be so obvious that stress can harm the heart. However, it is a well established risk factor, although many who lead stressful lives are not aware of it. They believe that being under pressure is good, and get hooked on it, learning to live with their poor sleeping habits and the constant feeling of tiredness. Of course the occasional periods of stress are unavoidable, and a healthy person can cope easily with them. What must be guarded against is constant poor sleep (or lack of it), tiredness, exhaustion, irritability, fear and anxiety. Sensible management of one's life along the lines suggested, especially aerobic exercise, careful diet, and relaxation methods, may help avoid heart problems, although this does require a positive effort. Changing long-established habits is not easy.

Coping with heart problems

Once one has a heart problem, rehabilitation may proceed along various lines. Drugs, exercise, stress reduction, and surgery may all be necessary. Medical opinion on all these methods varies – each has its advocate.

Many individuals who suffer a heart attack are in poor physical shape, and are nervous and fearful after release from hospital. Properly supervised exercise may help to prevent further attacks and prolong life, but it will certainly bring the individual back to a better physical condition (which is a good thing in itself) and also restore mental equilibrium. The individual will of course come under the supervision of his physician, but at some point he will be on his own again in familiar surroundings. Whatever he does must be gradually built up, starting from very low levels. The intensity of the exercise, as registered in the increased pulse rate, should never be beyond the percentage of the maximum heart rate which is recommended by the doctor.

Cardiac patients will usually be recommended to take exercise to increase cardiovascular endurance (aerobic/circulo-respiratory/endurance/stamina) such as walking, running, swimming and cycling. The heart rate will be taken carefully up to a prescribed level, and kept there for a set length of time. Other types of exercise – such as those which involve lifting heavy weights, sharp bursts of high activity or holding the breath and straining – are to be strictly avoided.

Of course, exercise will vary according to the condition of the person. Some may have to start an exercise programme with a few extremely light, slow movements, and others may finish it running the marathon. The heart rate is always the important determining factor.

Stress

In addition, the individual must learn to recognise when he is coming under stress, and then deliberately 'throttle back'. The symptoms are: poor sleep, bad temper, aggression, grumbling, longer work hours (but less achieved), minor sicknesses, frustration, rages, feelings of persecution by colleagues and their lack of cooperation, talking, smoking and drinking too much.

Lower back pain

Pain in the lower back or the lumbar spine is a condition that afflicts a great many people. Epidemiological studies have revealed that back pain afflicts between sixty and eighty per cent of the population in the Western world. Back ache ranks second to headache as the most common medical complaint. However, there is a good deal of popular confusion about the causes and treatment for this condition.

The lumbar spine is a complicated portion of the anatomy, and back pain may result from any one of a large number of possible malfunctions. Possible causes range from simple injuries, muscular spasms, wear and tear, depression, pregnancy, to tumors and infections. In many cases back pain will clear up with a few weeks' rest, but in cases of chronic and debilitating pain surgery may be indicated. Obviously, if the pain is persistent, expert medical attention will be required. However, if the back is treated carefully in work or play, a good deal of backache can be avoided.

The functioning unit of the spine consists of two adjacent vertebrae and their intervening soft tissues, ligaments, discs and muscles. All these possess nerves which, if damaged, transmit back pain. The spine itself is balanced and controlled by a complex series of muscles. Crucial to the spine's stability are the abdominal muscles, the erector spinae muscle which runs down the back of the spine, and the iliopsoas muscle which runs along the front of the spine from the lumbar area to just below the hip joint. Exercises for these muscles are described later.

Certain conditions are associated with the onset of back pain. Heavy physical work, static work postures, frequent bending and twisting, lifting and forceful movements, repetitive work (i.e. in an assembly line), vibrations and obesity are all likely to be followed by back pain.

In these situations some elementary back care is essential. Heavy physical work, whether it involves lifting or carrying, must be lightened. For example, if a 100 lb load of building materials has to be moved, it is better to make five trips carrying 20 lbs each time than two trips with 50 lbs, or even one trip with 100 lbs. The load that is carried must be comfortable and well within the strength capacity of the individual. The tendency to carry or lift close to the limits of one's strength must be continually avoided. The correct technique of lifting must also be followed. Weight should always be lifted close to the trunk, with the back held as erect as possible.

When the weight is on the floor or low down, bend the legs into a squatting or semi-kneeling position and raise the weight by straightening the legs and keeping the back straight. A common source of back injury is from a movement involving a lift and a twist. If it is not possible to avoid this movement, make sure it is done with very light loads.

Static work postures may be either sitting or standing. Sitting places more stress on the spine than standing, so if you have to sit for long periods it is essential to sit correctly in a good seat. The ideal seat is first of all an adjustable one. The height of the seat and the backrest should be adjustable to individual needs. The feet should be flat on the floor with the knees bent at an angle of ninety degrees and the thighs fully supported along their length. The backrest should be positioned at the point of greatest inward curvature, namely the lumbar spine, and should support the back at that point but also allow some movement backwards. Arm rests, swivel and wheels are useful extras. When sitting, rest on the buttock bones and carry your body vertically above them. Avoid rolling back on the buttocks. Even the perfect chair is no guarantee against back pain, especially if sitting for long hours. One way round this is to work standing up. There is no law that says you have to type sitting down, for example. Building special work tables involves additional cost but may be preferable to having to give up work because of back pain. Orientals who spend a lot of their time sitting on the floor or squatting seem to suffer far less from back pain. Try sitting cross-legged on the floor when working. Some experimentation with work top levels will be necessary and it may take a while to get used to the position. After a little perseverance you may find this preferable to sitting in a chair.

If you have to stand still for long periods, rest one leg on a low box. This is the principle adopted in stand bars. Most of the traditional establishments had a foot rail for the drinker to rest one foot on while he spent hours standing at the bar. This is ergonomically quite sound.

Vibration is another factor associated with back pain. This is most commonly experienced when driving, which combines with prolonged sitting, often in poorly designed seats. A rolled towel in the small of the back and support under the thighs can make the seat more comfortable and occasional breaks from driving can be taken to relieve cramped posture, but little can be done to avoid the vibration.

The lower back, like any other part of the body, should be used frequently through its full range of movement. Excessive movement or movement over a limited range will eventually cause pain. Work that involves excessive bending and twisting or repetitive cramped movement such as in an assembly line will eventually lead to trouble. The remedy is obvious – do not work any portion of the anatomy excessively, and if doing work of limited movement take a break every forty-five minutes or so and exercise the back gently in all directions for a few minutes.

Sudden forceful movement is often the cause of back injury. A stuck window which suddenly gives, or the quick jerking movement against something which refuses to move, often wrenches the back. Such movements are best avoided or done very carefully if unavoidable. There are several sports such as golf which require sudden movement. The answer to this if the player suffers from back pain is to improve your playing technique or give it up altogether.

Obesity is commonly associated with back pain. The slim erect body is somewhat like a flagpole where all the weight sits over the base. However, a large stomach upsets this balance and makes the lower back work harder to counterbalance the weight. Dieting is the answer to this particular problem. A slim body and frequent general exercise both go a long way to avoiding back pain. A weak or underused back is more likely to cause trouble than a strong well-exercised one.

A stiff back may eventually lead to back problems. People commonly accept the fact that they can barely touch their toes, or arch up from a front lying position, or twist round when in the driving seat. This stiffness is accepted as natural, yet there is no reason why it should be natural. Young children, dancers, yoga practitioners and Orientals develop a much greater range of free movement with careful exercise, and there is no reason why most people cannot free their backs. Yoga is an excellent way to loosen the back, but patience is required. It may take three or four months going to a class once or twice a week to see results (see page 146).

Daily back care

Here is a list of do's and don'ts to safeguard your back in common situations in the home.

1 When washing dishes or ironing, position one foot higher than the other such as on a low box.

2 Carry or lift babies close to the body.
3 Use a long-handled vacuum cleaner, or kneel on one knee when cleaning.
4 Do not bend over to make the bed. Kneel on the bed with one knee and use one arm to brace yourself.
5 Avoid long periods of bent-over work, such as gardening or vacuuming. If possible work for ten minutes, then come back to it an hour or so later.
6 When typing or at meetings avoid long periods of sitting. Get up at frequent intervals and move around. Similarly, break up long journeys in cars or planes.
7 If carrying a load in one hand, try to counterbalance the load with something in the other hand.
8 Do not do any vigorous back work first thing in the morning.
9 If jogging, wear proper jogging shoes and avoid hard surfaces.
10 Do not lift or hold out any weight at arm's length.
11 Avoid sleeping on the stomach. If you have to, place a cushion under the hips.
12 When resting the back, lie flat on your back and bend the legs. Try resting the lower legs and back of the knees on some cushions. This takes the strain off the psoas muscle.
13 When making love, choose a position that avoids undue strain of the lower back.

Treating back pain

If back pain suddenly strikes, the best immediate course of action is to take some aspirins and go to bed, unless you have trouble urinating or distinct weakness in the legs, in which case you should call a doctor straightaway.

In most cases the back will right itself in two to three weeks with sufficient rest. Aspirin, heat and massage to the afflicted area may also help. If the pain persists or gets worse, call a doctor. Depending on the amount of residual pain, you can gradually return to your normal schedule. However, if this involves any of the factors associated with back pain, such as static work postures or heavy physical work, you will have to use your ingenuity and limit these till you can get back into full stride.

Once you are free from pain, some simple exercises will help.

Exercises for the back

The spine is mainly supported by the two muscles which run down the sides of the spine at the back – the erector spinae, and the iliopsoas muscle which lies on the other side of the spine deep in the groin and hip. In addition the spine is supported by strong stomach muscles and abdominal pressure.

11.1 Sit-up

This is one of the best exercises for increasing stomach strength. However, care must be taken not to irritate the iliopsoas muscle. You can avoid this by sitting up with the knees bent. Sit-ups done with the legs straight or with the feet hooked under a fixed object work the psoas too hard (see page 182). Do the sit-ups with the arms folded across the chest, or with the hands clasped behind the head. Aim for twenty to twenty-five sit-ups, once or twice a day.

11.2 Stomach tensing

In this exercise the stomach is tensed hard. However, make sure that you close the anus and involve all the abdominal muscles. It can be done sitting or standing at virtually any time. Practise tensing the muscles fifteen to twenty times, holding the tension for no longer than a second or two, two or three times a day. Do not do this exercise if you have any of the coronary risk factors (see page 180).

11.3 Pelvic tilt

This is not an easy exercise to describe. Stand against a wall or lie on the floor. Between the wall or floor and your lower back there should be a gap. Practice flattening your lower back against the wall or floor by tilting the pelvis and genitals forward and up. This exercise works both the erector spinae and the iliopsoas muscles. Do it fifteen to twenty times once or twice a day.

11.4 Clasping knees to chest

This exercise stretches the lower back. Lie flat on the floor with the knees bent. First practise lifting one knee to the chest as near as you can get it, then pull it the rest of the way with two hands. Hold briefly in position then relax, return the leg to its original position, and repeat with the other leg. Eventually practise lifting both knees to the chest at the same time. Do this exercise about ten times, twice a day.

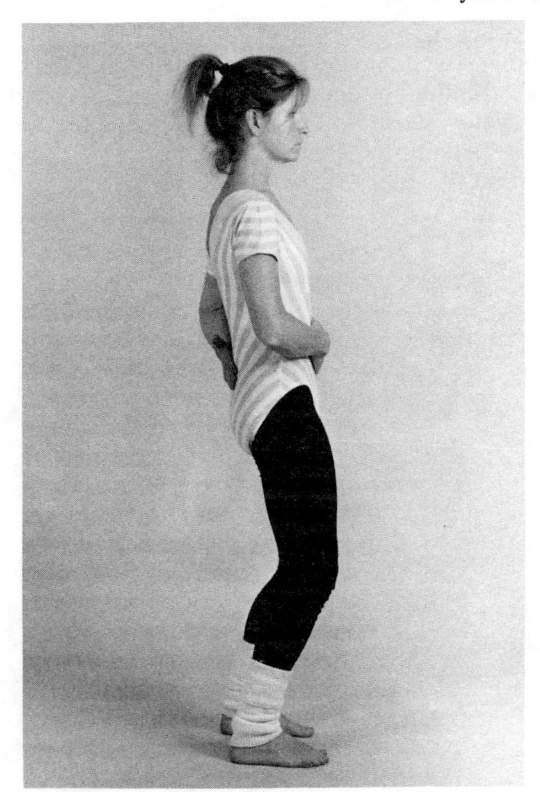

Exercise 11.3

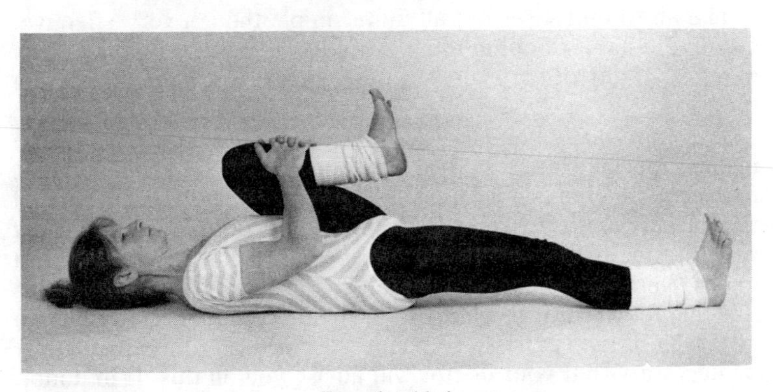

Exercise 11.4

11.5 Squat

This is another stretching exercise. Squat down, feet flat on the floor if possible, with the bottom as low as possible. Stay squatting for fifteen to twenty seconds. This position bends the spine in the opposite way to its customary inward curve.

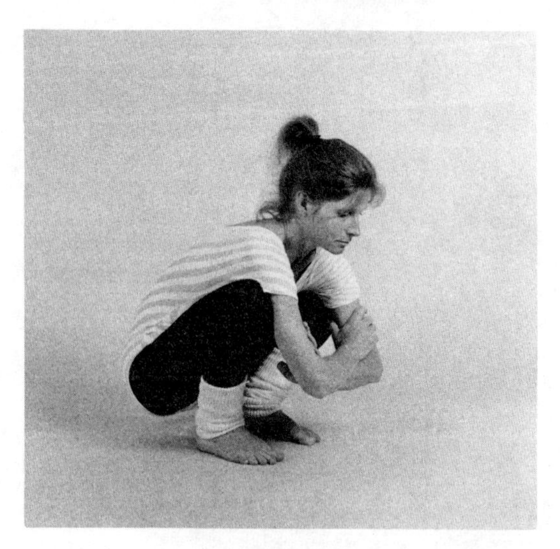

Exercise 11.5

The above exercises are all quite simple though very effective. Get in the habit of doing them every day – it will only take a few minutes. If any of the exercises cause more back pain, stop doing them.

There are many non-surgical ways of treating back pain. These include special exercises, yoga, spinal manipulation, acupuncture, massage, traction, corsets and plaster casts. The success rate of these treatments is between sixty and seventy per cent, and they are worth trying provided you have made sure you are in competent hands. Knowing about your back and basic back care as described in this chapter will also go a long way to help alleviate pain and avoid it generally. If pain persists, some invasive or surgical treatment may be necessary, but your doctor will advise you on this. If in doubt, you should get a second opinion.

12

Nutrition and Weight Loss

This chapter is mainly about losing weight. For many people, their chief interest in fitness is simply in *looking* fit, and more specifically in losing unsightly excess weight around the thighs, hips, stomach and upper arms. This is dealt with in some detail later, but first it is necessary to consider what is the right diet to rear and maintain a healthy body – which brings us to the science of nutrition.

The nutritional functions of food

Food has three main nutritional functions. It provides:

1 *Energy* (carbohydrates and protein);
2 Material for *building* and *repair* (protein);
3 Material for the *regulation* and *control* of energy, growth and repair (vitamins and inorganic materials).

Energy comes from fats, starches, proteins and sugars, and can be found in such foods as lard, butter, margarine, cheese, bacon, cereals, pasta, sugar, beans, peas, nuts, potatoes, and so on.

Building and repair materials are provided by protein, calcium, and iron, and are found in such foods as milk, cheese, eggs, meat, fish, cereals, peas, beans, and so on.

Regulation and control materials are calcium, iron, iodine, phosphorus and the vitamins, and can be found in milk, cheese, eggs, bacons, fatty fish, and some fruit and vegetables.

Except for a few man-made foods, no one item of food provides all the essentials; only a mixed diet can provide everything the body needs. However, there is not one 'right' diet which can provide all these essentials, but any number of possibilities. For example, all the essential requirements may be covered by a diet that is largely vegetarian, or by one that is largely derived from animal products.

In the richer countries of the world, the intake of energy, and building and repair foods is usually satisfactory, but the intake of control and regulation materials needs some attention. Since only some fruits and vegetables provide vitamins, one cannot assume that an indiscriminate visit to the greengrocer's shop will be enough. Children, and especially adolescents, require greater amounts of these materials than adults. In other words, there is an erratic distribution of vitamins among foods. Four common food items, however, belong to all three categories; namely, bacon, milk, cheese and fatty fish (such as herrings). These are readily available and fairly cheap, and a regular supply will help to make up for any general deficiencies.

A diet should not only be mixed in overall terms, but also on a meal-to-meal basis. That is to say, each meal should contain a combination of the types of food, especially the proteins and carbohydrates. Protein taken without carbohydrate is largely lost to the body. Thus it is wise to take rice and beans, or bread and cheese, or cereal and milk together in any one meal. The practice of having one very 'meaty' meal and another mainly of bread, as is sometimes the case in institutional cooking, should be avoided if possible.

Energy foods

Although many foods have a dual or even a triple nutritional function, the main requirement on a day-to-day basis is for energy production. Whereas the body can go without the other types of food for some time, it will soon notice a lack of energy. The body has to take in the 1 lb (½ kg) or so of food each day to keep moving, and the bulk of this has to be energy-producing food. This is most easily and cheaply provided by such foods as potatoes, beans, grain (such as bread and rice) and pasta (such as spaghetti). An animal protein such as meat does not have to provide the bulk of a meal, but can form quite a small proportion of it, or even be omitted as in the case of vegetarians, even though meat supplies a considerable amount of energy.

Protective foods

Our appetite will soon tell us whether we have had a sufficient amount of energy foods, but some time may elapse before the body shows evidence of the lack of the protective foods (inorganic materials and vitamins). The foods that protect the body from such diseases as rickets can be roughly grouped into the five categories shown below:

1 Dairy foods
2 Vegetables and fruit
3 Whole grain cereals
4 Liver and other offals
5 Fish and other sea produce

A sensible diet should first ensure that there is an adequate supply of these protective foods, with protein and energy requirements coming second and third. Unfortunately, people's diets are usually the other way round, with energy foods the main consideration, and the protective foods generally left to look after themselves. Cost and taste are of course major factors, but some effort should be made to eat such things as liver, fish, bacon and cheese regularly.

Foods with a high fibre content are also protective, but not quite in the same way. They include wholemeal bread, bran, baked beans, whole cereals, fruit and vegetables. A regular intake of such foods gives the intestines something to 'bite' on, and helps to avoid diseases such as diverticulitis. Also protective, but yet again in a different way, is a diet low in animal fats. A high level of blood fat is a risk factor in coronary disease, and this can be avoided by eating as little animal fat as possible. Fortunately there is no need to eat much of this food anyway, since the inorganic materials and vitamins that it provides are only needed in minute quantities. As mentioned above, the bulk of any diet should be energy foods such as bread and rice.

Dietary doctrine

Diet is a highly contentious subject. New 'facts' about food emerge almost every week, and fairly soon a dietary doctrine surrounds them. One does not have to look very far, however, to find someone who is an exception to almost any theory. An additional complication is that nutrition is not an exact science. It is fairly easy to spot some relationships, such as the link between scurvy and the lack of vitamin C, but extremely difficult to know what happens to the various chemicals we take in through our mouths when they merge into the vast melting pot of chemicals which is our body. The various possible interactions between these chemicals are countless. The best that one can do, perhaps, is to fulfill the known orthodox nutritional requirements as above, to avoid or minimise the intake of known toxic substances, and then to vary the choice of food as much as possible. In other words, when we are not too sure about the food we eat, we should take as wide a range as possible, and cook it in different ways. Then we are likely to get it right most of the time, and wrong not too often. This also applies when in doubt about the additives in processed and packaged foods. Eat as much fresh food as possible, and if it is impossible to avoid additives, vary the brands, so the additives differ.

Changing eating habits is as difficult as changing any other habit; however a start can be made by keeping a record for a few weeks of exactly what you eat, including any little snacks or drinks. At the end of this period look back, and see if you can detect any deficiencies or trends. It may be that you eat too much fried, tinned or packaged food, or of any one single food. Also check whether the vegetables you eat are raw or cooked, or whether you eat large quantities of refined foods, such as white bread, sugar and flour.

Sugar, especially white sugar, has been attacked on several counts. Firstly it is not strictly necessary. A diet without added sugar would be completely satisfactory, as all necessary energy can be taken from carbohydrates and fats. Next, sugar is responsible for the elevation of the blood sugar level, which can produce a swing between a feeling of 'quick energy' and lightheadedness. Thirdly, sugar elevates the blood triglycerides and may stimulate the liver to produce more cholesterol, both of which are recognised coronary risk factors. In addition, sugar, especially hidden sugar like that contained in chocolate, biscuits, cakes, cornflakes, ice-cream, soft drinks, jelly and fruit-flavoured yoghourt represents 'empty' calories. That is, it has no nutritional value and only provides unnecessary calories to add to the body's weight.

Other refined foods such as white flour and polished rice suffer in that the process of refinement removes not only the fibre, but other parts of nutritional value.

Finally, recent research has drawn attention to the link between salt and high blood pressure. Some experts have recommended a salt intake of no more than one to two teaspoonfuls per day.

Once you have an idea of your eating patterns, start to plan odd changes. Change the method of cooking from frying to boiling or steaming if you eat too many fried foods, or include some raw vegetables or fruit in the meal. Also use different proportions of proteins and carbohydrates, or try surviving on vegetarian meals for a day. The emphasis is of course on variety, and this can be carried through to the restaurant where you can make it a frequent practice to choose a dish you have never tried before, or to go to restaurants cooking food from different countries. It does not take much effort or imagination to vary your diet and food preparation.

Weight loss

For various reasons obesity is a widespread problem. Medically, the overweight are more likely to die younger and to suffer from such problems as high blood pressure. Visually, they are objects of fun in our society, which is increasingly orientated to slimness and fitness. Gross obesity is in itself an unpleasant condition, limiting the range and intensity of movement, and normal everyday activities such as climbing stairs. However, the overweight do not need to be told this, and judging by the amount of information on dieting that is always available, there are a considerable number of overweight people.

To a large extent, the bane of the overweight is the simplicity of the remedy. The lean say: eat less, or be more active, or do both. However, if it were as simple as this there would be very few overweight people around. The hidden assumption is that only will-power is required, and that if you cannot lose weight you are morally defective in some way. But food intake and physical activity are very difficult habits to change. Acquiring knowledge about nutrition and exercise, and then acting upon that knowledge requires effort, in some ways like learning a new sport. The more you learn and put into practice, the easier it becomes, until one day it is habitual, and there is no problem. When changing your eating and activity habits, various devices and strategems are needed to bridge the difficult early stage. The effort required in the early stages of changing your eating habits is not just physical; it is a more difficult kind of effort. It requires the denial of immediate pleasure (eating) for some future pleasure (looking slim and feeling fitter) via one major remedy (exercise) which is initially potentially uncomfortable. The problem is in bridging the pleasure gap. To lose weight, and stabilise your weight, it is necessary to:

1 Set goals;
2 Understand weight gain and loss;
3 Act upon facts about nutrition and persevere.

Setting goals

Setting goals requires an estimate of how overweight you are, and then the ability to measure change as you grow slimmer. Although the bathroom mirror may show a person that he is too fat, it is more likely that the scales will be used as the main indicator. There is a difference, however, between being heavy and too fat. A body builder who builds up an enormous amount of extra muscle will certainly be much heavier than standard ideal height and weight tables will indicate for a person of his height.

The first thing to do is to get an historical profile of your shape. Look out old holiday snaps or even childhood photographs, and try to get an idea of the change in your shape. If there has been change it is possible to change back, but sometimes there may not have been change. At this point it is wise to make sure that you are not trying to change into a shape you will never achieve. Some people may have carried an ideal shape in their heads since childhood which in no way corresponds to their own potential, for example a large-boned woman who has always wanted to be slim and model-like. You should also have a clear idea of your present shape, so you could get someone to take up-to-date photographs of yourself from different angles just dressed in swimwear. These can be used to compare with past and future pictures as you battle to lose weight. As an alternative to this, you could try making a video recording of yourself.

Next, take all the measurements you can. Use a tape measure to measure your waist, thighs, hips, upper arms and so on. It is possible for you to become slimmer as sagging muscles are toned up, but still remain the same weight. The tape measure and your clothing sizes will show this progress even when the scales do not.

Since overall bodyweight is not the only indicator of obesity try the skinfold test. The overweight person really needs to get rid of *fat*, and this can be measured where it lies under the skin. Special callipers are needed to do the job properly and measurements should be taken all over the body – however, as a rough rule of thumb, anything over an 'inch of pinch' is too fat. Use your thumb and forefinger to gather in a large fold of skin and fat and check to see if it is over an inch thick between the fingers. Suitable areas to measure are the stomach, and the backs of the upper arms and thighs.

Having surveyed the problem, you need to estimate an ideal weight. Insurance company tables which give an ideal weight based on age, height and sex are useful for this. Often the weights will be given for people of small, medium and large frames. Beware of underestimating your ideal weight, as if your target is set too low, you will have real trouble in meeting it. Unrealistic expectations more often than not lead to breakdowns in the reducing programme. Having selected a target weight, simple arithmetic will give a figure of how many pounds or kilos need to be lost. The next danger is deciding on an unrealistic rate of fat loss. Those who go for massive and rapid loss of weight frequently give up, and then compensate for their subsequent feelings of inadequacy by overeating heavily. Their life becomes a yo-yo between periods of fasting and binging, with depression in between and no overall decrease in body fat. A simple target of one or two pounds a week is not too difficult to achieve, and is easily estimated in relation to food intake and exercise.

Understanding weight gain and loss

Having gathered all the measurements and set realistic goals, the next stage is to understand the relevant facts about weight gain and loss. The body gains extra weight (fat) by taking in more energy in food than it expends in activity. Both energy intake and energy expenditure can be calculated in terms of calories. Thus there are three main lines of attack. Fat can be trimmed off by reducing the amount of food eaten, or by becoming more active, or by doing both at the same time. The third method appears to have the best rate of success.

Many overweight people protest that they eat very little, and this may well be true. Studies show that although the overweight often eat very little, they are also usually very inactive. Thus the equation stays the same – their energy expenditure is less than their energy intake, and so they get fatter.

Dieting is probably the most popular method of weight control, and exercise the least. Many of the overweight criticise exercise on various grounds. Often it is pointed out that a pound of fat, for example, is equivalent to 3500 calories, and that to lose that in exercise alone, it would be necessary to walk for twelve hours or to bicycle for nine. This is true, but ignores the fact that exercise has a cumulative effect. In the same way that fat is put on slowly, so it can be taken off slowly, a small amount at a time, with the help of exercise. A brisk walk for half an hour every day over a period of three years would take off an enormous amount of fat. Another criticism of exercise is that it only increases the appetite. This is not necessarily true. Exercise in periods lasting between thirty and sixty minutes can lessen the appetite. Also it has been found that the quantity of food eaten by the inactive overweight is very similar to that eaten by very active, slim people. Exercising will not necessarily increase food intake beyond that of the very active.

Some overweight people also criticise exercise as being difficult to compute in terms of calorie expenditure, but most activities now have calorie ratings. The final accusation is that exercise is harmful, and may cause you to drop dead from a heart attack. Everyone has their limits, beyond which exercise can be harmful, but a careful build-up within these limits is quite safe. More people die in bed than elsewhere, but it is not suggested that we avoid going to bed!

For those who rely solely on restricting the amount of food taken, there is a whole host of measures, of which calorie counting is the most popular. There is a significant variation in the amount of calories an individual needs – for example, growing children need more calories per pound of bodyweight than adults. One method of estimating your own requirements is to multiply your pre-dieting weight (in pounds) by 7 and by 15, and select a figure between the two. A 150 lb (70 kg) adult would therefore need somewhere between 1050 and 2250 calories per day. The lower figure would certainly result in weight loss and the higher one in some weight gain. Since it is difficult to be exact, the actual number of calories taken per day would have to be varied over a period to find the figure that results in loss. Another method is to equate one pound of fat with 3500 calories, which means that a reduction of 500 calories per day would result in a loss of one pound body fat per week.

To count calories, you have to know how many calories any particular item of food (and drink) contains. Pocket guides with this information are readily available. Various diets are popular at any time, such as the carbohydrate restricted diet and the high fibre diet, but it is probable that the diet which is most likely to succeed is the one that is closest to your present eating habits, and that requires a cutting back of what you eat already rather than switching to a completely different type of food regime.

Instead of counting calories, an effective way to lose weight is by cutting out certain foods. Desserts can quite easily be eliminated from meals, as can second helpings. Cutting out tea and coffee, especially if taken with cream and sugar, can show a quick weight loss. When you feel like a cup of coffee or tea, take a drink of water instead. Quite often it is simple thirst that prompts the feeling for tea and with a glass of water the feeling passes. This is easier to do in the summer. Many other items such as biscuits, cakes, chocolates, sweets, peanuts, crisps, fizzy drinks and alcohol can be ruthlessly pruned from your diet. A look at your normal diet will show a preponderance of any single item and cutting this out may tip the balance towards leanness.

A loss of 500 calories per day can be achieved by a *decrease* of 250 calories in food intake combined with a 250 *increase* in calories consumed by exercise, or any ratio of food decrease and exercise increase equivalent to 500 calories. This represents a fat loss of 1 lb per week. To lose 2 lbs a week, which is still realistic and not too drastic, the daily figure is double, namely 1000 calories. Exercise does not have to be continuous, of course. Half an hour's walk in the morning and back in the evening will burn up roughly 200 calories (depending on speed), and any other more vigorous activity during the day, such as climbing stairs, will add to the total.

On the food side of the equation, 250 calories could be saved by *not* consuming one cup of coffee with cream and sugar, two plain biscuits and an apple. It can be seen that the food reduction is not enormous, especially when it is combined with a little extra physical activity. Provided you are content to make slow progress, a loss of 1 lb per week represents 52 lbs (24 kg) in a year, which is significant.

Acting upon the information

Armed with information about the basic equation for weight loss, the next stage is to put it into operation. First, you need to gather together all the necessary equipment, such as scales, tape measures, food tables and so on. Next, you must take all possible measurements, and some photographs. To know if you are losing weight or getting thinner, you must have some means of comparison. Thirdly, you must have information about what you eat and how active you are. This may well come as a bit of a shock. If you faithfully record exactly what you eat and how much exercise you take over a week, the picture that emerges may well contradict your fond image of yourself. In addition to recording everything that you eat and drink, it is essential to record the time and situation in which it happened. A lot of extra food often depends on the social setting, for example, if a friend pops round for a chat, or you go out for a drink after work. In such cases it is often easier to cut out the socialising than to continue to socialise and cut down on what you take. Another example is having food on display in the house. If you find that a lot of your snacks consist of helping yourself from a box of chocolates or a bowl of peanuts, then take the simple step of not displaying the food. A very careful examination of your eating habits often reveals eating situations which can easily be avoided.

A similar investigation of your daily activities will also reveal opportunities for additional exercise, for example walking to the shops instead of driving, or not taking the lift for one or two floors.

Best of all, try to make time for regular walks, rides, swims, runs, dances, and exercise classes. Any exercise tends to increase the body's metabolic rate for a while, and the increased metabolic rate can be maintained with regular periods of activity.

Having found your opportunities for food-loss and activity-gain, make use of them, and *record* them. This is important. A loss of a pound of fat a week is not spectacular; you will need all the evidence of progress that you can gather, to sustain your drive. Even a small recorded weight loss may increase your enthusiasm, and push you on.

There will inevitably be set-backs on either front. A celebration of some sort may put on a pound or two, and a cold may stop activity for two weeks. Progress in the first few weeks may be small, especially if you are exercising a lot, as there may be some muscle gain as well as fat loss. In this situation, the tape measure rather than the scales will show a decrease in your size. If you do have set-backs, try to recoup the ground you have lost – and here records are vital.

Help from friends or family is invaluable. Tell them what you are doing, and get them to praise all your achievements – but do not make a weight-loss an excuse for a family celebration!

It may be that you are drawn irresistibly to certain foods, in which case there are other methods to help you. One is to imagine the food, then to imagine worms in it, or yourself vomiting after eating it. Another useful method is relaxation and meditation. Where the urge to eat stems from anxiety, tension or fear, controlling this will help to control your food intake. A reduction in weight is frequently reported by women who regularly do yoga, for example, although the actual amount of calories expended is very small. Very relaxed people often find it easy to resist food in the form of snacks or extra helpings or drinks. Eating when not hungry is disturbing to their relaxed equilibrium. Relaxation and exercise may both work because they put you in touch with yourself.

Despite all the information and advice on weight loss, it remains a problem to many, and it is not fully clear why this should be so. However, one thing is obvious, and that is that the various remedies all require effort in one form or another. Whatever effort you have to make must become habitual, since your ideal weight should be maintained for the rest of your life. You must adopt attitudes to food and exercise which will last a lifetime. Whatever tactics you choose, ask yourself if you can continue this for the rest of your life.

Bearing this in mind, avoid drastic diets and harsh exercise regimes; when you fail you will probably blame yourself, and go on a binge to console yourself. Think of the process of changing your attitudes to food and exercise as resembling that of turning an enormous ship around – it has to be done slowly, a few degrees at a time.

Further Reading

Astrand and Rodahl, *Textbook of Work Physiology* (McGraw Hill Book Co., New York, 1978).

R. A. Berger, *Applied Exercise Physiology* (Lea and Febiger, Philadelphia, 1982).

K. Cooper, *Aerobics* (Bantam Books, New York, 1968).

M. Dena Gardiner. *Principles of Exercise Therapy*, 4th ed. (Bell and Hyman, London, 1980).

J. Goodbody and Kirkley (eds), *Manual of Weight Training* (Stanley Paul, London, 1982).

Sophy Hoare, *Tackle Yoga* (Stanley Paul, London, 1982).

B. K. S. Iyengar, *Light on Yoga*, 2nd ed. (Allen and Unwin, London, 1971).

M. D. LeBow, *Weight Control* (John Wiley, Chichester, 1981).

Trevor Leggett, *Chapter of the Self* (Routledge and Kegan Paul, London, 1978).

Mathen and Halhuber (eds), *Controversies in Cardiac Rehabilitation* (Springer-Verlag, 1982).

A. Maxwell, I. Burdon, S. McDonald, *Faber's Anatomical Atlas* (Faber and Faber, London, 1962).

L. Morehouse, *Physiology of Exercise*, 7th ed. (CV Mosby, St Louis, 1976).

L. Morehouse and L. Gross, *Total Fitness in Thirty Minutes a Week* (Granada, London, 1977).

R. F. Mottram, *Human Nutrition*, 4th ed. (Edward Arnold, London, 1981).

Bill Tancred and Geoff Tancred, *Weight Training for Sport* (Hodder and Stoughton, Sevenoaks, 1984).

Bruce Tulloh, *Natural Fitness* (Arrow Books, London, 1976).

Augustus A. White, *Your Aching Back* (Bantam Books, London, 1983).

John Yudkin, *This Slimming Business*, 4th ed. (Penguin, London, 1974).